TOUGH CARE

*Never stop caring no matter
how tough it gets*

Bernard Mooney

ISBN-10: 1466391375
ISBN-13: 9781466391376

Library of Congress Control Number: 2011918003
CreateSpace, North Charleston, SC

In Memoriam

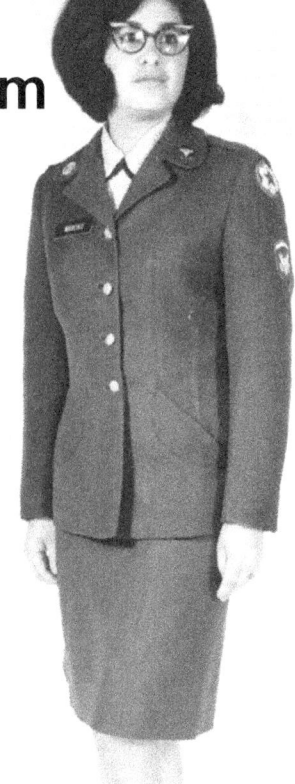

Celia (Mendez) Mooney
1944–2010

US Army Women's Army Corps
1964–1972

Contents

Introduction   vii

Chapter One—She Is Gone   1

Chapter Two—Tough Care Journal Begins   7

Chapter Three—Caring for the
Caregiver—Yourself   25

Chapter Four—Endurance   33

Chapter Five—Control   45

Chapter Six—The Beginning of the End   51

Chapter Seven—Professional Help with
Tough Care   57

Chapter Eight—The End State   65

Chapter Nine—Respect from la Familia   71

Chapter Ten—Taps   79

Chapter Eleven—Lessons Learned   85

Afterword   99

Appendix A—The Mourner's Bill of Rights   99

           (Reprinted with permission)

Appendix B —Arlington National
  Cemetery Burial Eligibility   103

Appendix C—Pallas Athena(Reprinted
  with permission)   109

Appendix D—History of the Women's
  Army Corps
           (Reprinted with permission)   113

Appendix E—Some Useful Online Resources   119

Acknowledgments   123

References   125

Introduction

I am going to use the introduction of this book to answer two fundamental questions:

Why am I writing this book?

Why should you read it?

I just spent four years caring for my wife of thirty-nine years and watching while she died very slowly and painfully before my eyes. I took the best care of her that I could. I did it almost entirely on my own. As with most of our time together, it was she and I together against the odds. Telling our story should be a catharsis for me. That is to say, I am going to express all of the very difficult thoughts, feelings, and experiences that I have been through over the past four years. Expressing myself is said to be the same as expelling these thoughts, feelings, and experiences so as to relieve myself from the burdens that they place upon me. Put more simply, I need to get some stuff off my chest.

You should read this story because I am a baby boomer, as you might be as well. I was born in 1951, and there are many other baby boomers among you out there who might benefit from my experiences over the past few years. I was my lifelong mate's lone caregiver for all but a few weeks of her last years on this earth. During those last several weeks, I was still her primary caregiver with assistance from home nursing and home hospice professionals. The process of her illness and subsequent passing was long, painful, and arduous for us both. I believe that you may benefit from reading about what that process entailed for us. I doubt that anyone's future experience would exactly match the situation that she and I recently went through together. However, her illnesses related to diabetes, hypertension, stroke, dementia, and depression are illnesses that are rather common among us all. It is predictable that many people will face very similar circumstances that she and I faced together over the past several years. It is unfortunate, and inevitable, that the ending will be the same.

There are academic and industry studies that have determined that home care has been more prevalent than one might imagine in the US. It would appear that nearly a third of American households had someone who has served as a family caregiver within the last twelve months. This would indicate that tens of millions of families include at least one home caregiver.

It then stands to reason that as the baby boom generation ages over the next few decades, the numbers of folks needing care can only increase, exponentially. The actuarial tables also show that the quantity of younger people available to provide care will decline. This means that future caregivers will be older, on average. They will likely have infirmities of their own, as well.

Now you know why I'm writing this story. It is based upon one selfish reason and another reason not so selfish. After you have finished reading the book, we will both know whether or not my purposes were achieved.

Chapter One

She is Gone

She is finally, mercifully gone.
It is Tuesday, November 9, 2010.

Celia's last years were pure misery for her. Her Women's Army Corps (WAC) ethos did not abide by someone helping her to do everything, every day (not even her husband of thirty-nine years). Her mentality and her spirit were those of Athene the Greek warrior goddess. Athene was the ancient Greek goddess of wisdom and battle. She represented battle with intelligence and wisdom behind it, not just war for war's sake. The weak, helpless, and mostly paralyzed state Celia had been in for four years hurt her ten times as much as it might hurt someone else. She lived in misery every moment of every day of those years. She had been my mate and the mother of my children for thirty-nine years, and she was gone to her Maker.

I found her this morning lying in her hospital bed right next to our marriage bed, where I now slept alone. She lay there with eyes wide open, but not seeing. Her facial expression was quiet, peaceful, and relaxed. Gone were the tight wrinkles of pain in her forehead. Gone was the sad confusion in her eyes. I knew then what they meant when they talked about the sightless eyes of the dead. She was warm to the touch. Her limbs were loose, flexible, and relaxed. The night before, her legs were constricted in a rigid, bent, painful position.

At first I thought she might have awakened a little early—it was about 8:00 am. That was not the case. I spoke to her several times but got no response. Recently her responses were limited to grunts or shakes of the head. None of those were forthcoming. The last actual words she spoke to me a few days earlier were "you son of a bitch, you bastard." As I will discuss a little later in the story, there might be several possible explanations for this.

By about 8:15 am, it finally struck me that this might be it. After four long years of wondering, then dreading and then anticipating it, death had finally come for her. I remembered that during the wee hours of the morning—around three or four am—I had been awakened by a change in her breathing pattern. I had been forewarned by the hospice case manager/nurse that there was a specific breathing pattern called Cheyne-Stokes Syndrome that would mean that she was entering her final weeks and days. Last night was the first time I noticed it, and it preceded her passing by hours at the most. At the same time as her breathing changed, I saw what appeared to be three small luminous globes about the size of a tennis ball. They spun upward in a spiral pattern and disappeared through the bedroom ceiling. I was only partly awake and assumed that I was just seeing things and forgot about it. I am not particularly religious, but I saw what I saw. I will leave its real meaning and interpretation to you and your own beliefs about death and the period that may or may not follow it.

Nobody is ever prepared to deal with the death of someone close, no matter how long it might have been expected. I was not ready, even though I had by then been discussing her imminent demise on a daily basis with more than a dozen nurses/assistants for almost a month. Somehow, none of the physicians whom she saw regularly over a period of years had ever even mentioned the word *terminal*. In fairness to them, neither she nor I had ever asked.

I realized that I needed to do the right thing and quickly. Part of signing up to the home hospice agreement was that you agree not to call 911 in the event of apparent death and call the home hospice twenty-four-hour number instead. This was based on the fact that the home hospice agreement included a formal and legally binding "Do Not Resuscitate," or DNR, order.

I could not feel any pulse in her neck or in her wrist, but I wanted to convince myself that I would not be crying wolf. I took her temperature orally and it was 96.2, twice in a row. I recalled an old trick of putting a mirror under the nostrils of someone who you thought might be dead. The mirror did not fog at all.

I had watched her energetic vibrancy wane over the last four years, just as the harvest moon wanes in the sky over the course of a month. Now it was gone forever. It would not return to repeat its cycle the way the moon does.

I called the home hospice call center. They said a duty nurse would come as soon as possible. The on-call nurse showed up within the hour. She confirmed that Celia was gone. She said the condition of her pupils indicated that it had been another stroke. It would have been number four or five. The exact number of strokes she had suffered was unclear. She also suffered an uncountable number of TIAs (Transient Ischemic Attacks). These were micro-strokes that occurred without apparent symptoms. Their aggregate impact could total to the equivalent of a significant stroke. It would now be a distinction without a difference. It clearly did not matter anymore. Her extreme mental, emotional, and physical suffering was all over.

In addition to the formal declaration of death and its time, the nurse and I had to witness and sign documents concerning the destruction (flushing) of all remaining hard narcotics that were in the house from her care. That included small quantities of methadone and instant-release morphine that I had not yet administered. The hospice staff contacted a local funeral home, which retrieved Celia from the house within an hour or two. While I waited, I thought back two evenings prior. As I gave her last daily dose of morphine, she stared up at me with such sad, resigned eyes. I asked her, "You are going, aren't you?" She gave no discernable reply—neither word nor gesture. I reminded her that her boys and her baby sister were going to come and see her in a matter of days. Again, there was no reaction. I believe she knew it was her time. She knew that for her death would equal comfort, finally.

By odd coincidence, I had stopped at the funeral home the day prior. Based on all the time estimates I had discussed with the nurses who supervised her care over the last few weeks, I went in thinking that I probably had only a few months before I would need their services. I picked up some general brochures, price lists, and the business card of one of the funeral directors. I couldn't know at the time that they would be at my home the very next day.

As the funeral home staff took her, they asked me if I wanted to retain the rings she was wearing. I absentmindedly said to leave them on her. This was an error I would later correct.

Her death marked the end of an arduous four-year period of attending to her that I have come to call *tough care*.

Chapter Two

A Tough Care Journal Begins

You have probably heard of tough love. If you are a parent, you may have practiced it in one form or another. You may have had it practiced upon you as a child or teenager.

Beginning in early 2007, I became engaged in something similar that I called tough care. The tough in tough care did not describe toughness on the part of the caregiver, but rather the tough circumstances under which the caregiver had to continue to care (in every sense of that word) for a loved one.

March 2007 — *I have become responsible for the care of my wife of thirty-nine years. She needs care because she has suffered two strokes, numerous TIAs (Transient Ischemic Attacks), and has serious neuropathy caused by type II diabetes that was not properly treated over a period of years. She is deeply depressed as well.*

I reflected back to when those thirty-nine years began. We met in Heidelberg, Germany, in 1971, when we were both stationed there in the Army. When we met, she outranked me by one grade (for a while). She was a staff sergeant E-6 and I was a specialist five (E-5). She was to be assigned to our battalion. She arrived during the Christmas holidays in 1971. When she arrived, I was the senior person on duty because most of the staff was on a relaxed holiday schedule. I was single and was assigned to cover the office, so the married folks could spend more time at home with their families. She reported during the middle of the afternoon. I received her paper orders and let her know that the next step in her process of reporting was to go to our higher headquarters in Schwetzingen, about 12 miles away. She asked what transportation might be available for her. The battalion commander's driver was hanging around in the office with nothing to do, since the commander had gone home to the states for Christmas with his family. I had him give SSG Celia Mendez a ride to the next stop on her path, and then return her to the WAC barracks for the night. She later told me that she was very impressed by the fact that a young, spunky E-5 had a driver at his disposal. She thought that, as an E-6, she would probably have something even better. This did not turn out to be true, of course.

As often happened in these situations, the officers at higher headquarters noticed that SSG Mendez was an attractive young woman,, and they changed her orders to have her assigned there, rather than to our battalion. It didn't matter, because the only place that WACs could live in that area of Germany was in Heidelberg, within walking distance of where I worked and lived.

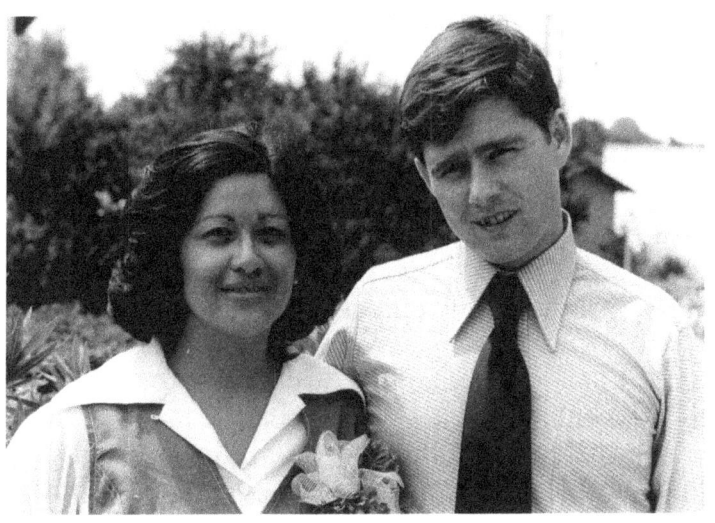

Celia and Bernie in Heidelberg, Germany, in the spring of 1972

As you might imagine, our current dire situation did not develop overnight. My wife suffered a major stroke in September 2005. The consensus of the doctors who treated her at the time was that the stroke would not create any long-term damage.

In June 2006, we flew the family over to Crete and attended our older son's wedding to a really great young lady he met while they were both pursuing graduate degrees in Architecture at Catholic University in Washington, DC. Celia was starting to have difficulty walking any great distance. She also had a few embarrassing episodes of incontinence, including one at the wedding reception. I opted to book her flight to include wheelchair assistance. It was a good thing I did. JFK alone would have been impossible without it. The Athens airport was no breeze either. Wheelchair passengers were deplaned in Athens using one of those food-catering trucks that elevates to the plane's galley. However, we all thoroughly enjoyed the fine wedding in Crete.

I reflected back to our own wedding. We wed in a small chapel on the outskirts of Heidelbeg in the spring of 1972. Our parents and families were not able to join us in Europe, so it was a small, informal affair. Poor Celia did not even understand what the priest was saying most of the time. He reverted to English for the important and legally binding questions. Our belated honeymoon took place in the late summer/early fall of 1972. We cruised most of the hot spots of Germany, Austria, Switzerland, Italy, France, and Spain in a 1969 Mustang coupe. The cover photo of this book shows Celia in front of the Eiffel tower in Paris toward the end of that trip.

A few weeks after returning from Scott and Ellie's wedding in Crete in 2006, I got a call at work from Celia's internist's office that she had been involved in an accident in their parking lot. I dashed over there and found an Alexandria, Virginia, police officer sitting in his cruiser at the entrance to the parking lot. I said, "Officer, I was told my wife was in a fender bender here. Do you know anything about that?" He replied in a rather deadpan way, "It was more than a fender bender, and they are all right over there."

Sure enough, Celia had managed to hit three other cars that were parked in the handicapped section of the parking lot. Fortunately it all happened at a pretty slow speed and no one was injured. She was pretty shook up, but not hurt in any way. She remembered nothing of what happened. As best we could determine, she thought the gearshift was in reverse when it was actually in drive. She looked out the back window and pressed the gas, but went forward into the other parked cars rather than back.

In December 2006, we left our home of twenty years in Virginia and moved to Las Vegas, Nevada — the land of high desert and rugged mountains.

I cashed out my half of the small company I had founded with a partner sixteen years earlier. We sold our half-acre home in northern Virginia. We gave away tons of stuff to neighbors. We left our two sons and their new families, careers, and lives behind.

It seemed like the right thing to do at the time, as they say. Celia had followed me around for over thirty years in the military and after. She had raised two boys almost single-handedly due to my frequent absences. As far as I was concerned, I owed her. If she wanted to return to her beloved southwest and to her extended family there, I felt she deserved to do so. I had completed a twenty-year army career. I had founded a successful small business and enjoyed the monetary and egotistical fruits of those endeavors. It was her turn to get whatever she wanted from life. Little did I know at the time that her obsessive insistence on moving to Las Vegas was actually an early instance of the insidious dementia that was just beginning to develop in her brain. It would be nearly a year later that I realized that her irrational and emotional need to move back to her roots was a symptom rather than just a strong desire.

We bought a spacious one-story, ranch-style house in the very new and upper-middle-class suburbs northwest of the infamous Las Vegas strip. Our older son, Scott, helped us pick it out from among ten we toured on a long weekend house-hunting trip on August 2006. Scott is an architect and interior designer. Scott's advice and opinions were very valuable in the house-hunting process.

On our drive out from Virginia, Celia was excited about the idea of reuniting with her extended family in and around Las Vegas. Her younger sister Belia had lived in Vegas for over twenty years. Belia's husband was a longtime floor man (you might know it as pit boss) at the Circus Circus casino. He had forty years on the job there. He knew all the names and some of the faces that we all heard about from the mobster days in Vegas. Celia also had aunts, uncles, cousins, and so forth, in some considerable numbers. They lived in and around Vegas or in Utah or California. Her emotional excitement was tempered, however, by some irksome physical impediments that we dealt with as best we could during the drive west. These centered on what appeared to us to be a balance problem when she walked, along with some occasional incontinence.

We moved into our new home in northwest Las Vegas in December 2006. The house is located on the slope of the Spring Mountain range on the west side of the Las Vegas Valley. It is at three thousand feet above sea level (as compared to sixteen hundred feet for the Las Vegas strip). The view is an impressive one in all directions. Mountains, desert, verdant valley, and the brightly lit strip are all so close you think you can touch them.

On that very day, Celia stumbled and fell while walking around our new back patio with her sister. Her cane got caught on the edge of the patio, and she fell pretty hard against the brick landscaping wall. That generated the first in a series of several emergency room visits we would have over the next few years.

The emergency room admission nurse very bluntly asked her if I had struck her to cause her injury. Celia defended me and told the nurse that a simple balance problem had caused her to stumble. Fortunately, her sister was with us and also made it clear that I had not been anywhere near them when Celia accidentally fell.

I started to wonder if she had some form of dementia. It was not yet clear whether it was Alzheimer's (early onset in her case) or some other variety. Her symptoms were nonspecific. Her near-term memory was measured in increments of minutes, rather than hours or days. She had no idea as to our address or phone number. She was completely unable to learn them. She was never sure what day, week, month, or year it was. Sometimes she remembered what city and state we were in, sometimes not.

Her long-term memory also started to deteriorate. She no longer had any idea of her age. It was sixty-three at that time.

Once, recently, she asked me to run out and get her some fresh fruit Danish for breakfast. I obliged and was gone about twenty-five minutes. When I returned, she angrily demanded to know why I brought Danish and where I had been. She then angrily demanded that I make her a ham sandwich. This incident caused me to make up some computer-printed reminder signs that I left in front of her from then on whenever I went out for short periods to take care of necessities. They said, in large bold font, where I was, and that I would be back soon.

May 2007 —*Tough care, like tough love, is caring for someone under some really tough circumstances. Physically, my wife has partial use of one arm, and that is about it. Her legs are less than 20 percent effective because of neuropathy. Neuropathy has damaged her nervous system. It stems, in her case, from diabetes. The neuropathy also causes her to be incontinent both in terms of urination and bowel movements. This contributes greatly to the reason I see this as tough care.*

We had moved just six months prior, but our shared wanderlust started to raise its adventurous head. We decided to make a trip that we both had talked about for years. It would be a train trip. We considered excursions through the northwest US and Canada. We finally decided to kill two birds with one stone. We would travel back east to see our two boys near Washington, DC, via train. Celia would need to be in a wheelchair for most of the way. It turned out that boarding a train with handicapped assistance and long-term parking support required traveling by car from Las Vegas to Union Station in Los Angeles.

We boarded the California Zephyr on Tuesday afternoon. As we waited I noticed that there was a group of travel trailers parked around the station. They all said House on them. I finally realized that an episode of the medical series with the grumpy doctor was filming there. I also then noticed how familiar the overall appearance of the station and its retro furnishings appeared to me, even though

I had never been there before. It has been a background character in any number of films and television episodes.

Our trip took us through the lower Rocky Mountains, but in the middle of the night. We weren't able to see much at all. We slept fitfully in our little sleeper compartment as the train jostled through the dark passes, tunnels, and raised trestles. The next day we were able to see our entry onto the broad plains of eastern Colorado and then Kansas. Celia preferred to remain seated in our compartment, while I occasionally ventured up to the observation car. It afforded a great view in every direction. A very supportive steward helped us by bringing us our meals from the dining car. The narrow passageway actually helped us quite a bit when it was time for her to visit the lavatory. She was still able to walk the short distance with my help.

We changed trains in Chicago two days after leaving LA. The Chicago-to-Washington leg was done in a day. We didn't recognize much, until we got pretty close to Union Station in Washington, DC. It seemed to us that the LA-to-Chicago part of the trip was in full HDTV color, while the Chicago-to-DC part presented itself on an old-fashioned, black-and-white television.

On the return trip to LA, our train was stopped by a derailment on the track ahead of another train. We stopped in Dodge City, Kansas. Wyatt Earp's statue adorned the city park. His Colt Peacemaker was drawn and aimed at the passing vehicle traffic.

The train crew was generally helpful and polite, but the central dispatchers who arranged bus transport from Dodge City to the next open station in Colorado forgot to consider the disabled folks on the train. There were four couples with wheelchair-bound travelers. Most of the passengers loaded straightforwardly onto three or four buses. I pointed out to a steward that none of the buses appeared to have any way of boarding a wheelchair. He assured me that proper transport would be arriving soon. He then scurried off with his cell phone held tightly to his ear. After a while, two minivans showed up from a local limousine service. They still had no special wheelchair accommodations, but at least there were no steps required to transfer our disabled companions into the vans. We then caught up with the others at the new train and resumed our travel without incident.

By the time we returned from the train trip, I realized that another part of the reason I saw this experience as tough care was psychological, on my part. I had abandoned all other pursuits in order to care for my wife. I shopped, cooked (rather poorly), cleaned, and washed. I did everything for us that we both had done together for a lot of years. I finally engaged a part-time respite care helper. Respite care provided assistance to me, the primary caregiver, so that I could get a break from the constant pressures and stresses of the work of caring for someone else. I used the respite care assistant to stay with Celia, while I left the house to perform necessary errands and tasks. I also had my own occasional medical appointments, haircuts, and other personal errands. This lady graciously also helped with the housekeeping and cooking. By the way, at this point there was no financial support from any government or medical insurance program with regard to Celia's care. This was true even though between us we had three forms of medical insurance.

Cooking was a real sore point. Celia's morale visibly collapsed when she realized she could no longer prepare a meal. She was renowned among family and friends everywhere for her cooking skills. Her Cinco de Mayo dinner parties were legend. There was nothing that she could not prepare, and prepare well. Her Mexican family background, together with our wide travels and diverse group of friends, caused our boys to grow up with a wide and varied exposure to different cuisines. She could master any line of food preparation from her native Hispanic foods, to oriental dishes she learned from friends, to a great old-fashioned red-blooded American potato salad.

Our younger son, Sean, is a successful professional chef. He attributes his vocation to his mom. He now owns a very eclectic set of cookbooks that Celia and I collected form many locations and many cultures.

I started my new role as a caregiver after completing a full twenty-year career in the army. I enlisted as an E-1 in 1970 with a high school diploma. I retired in 1990 as a major with an MBA. I then founded a small

computer-engineering firm in northern Virginia together with a partner. We ran the firm profitably for
sixteen years. It was a good gig that paid well.

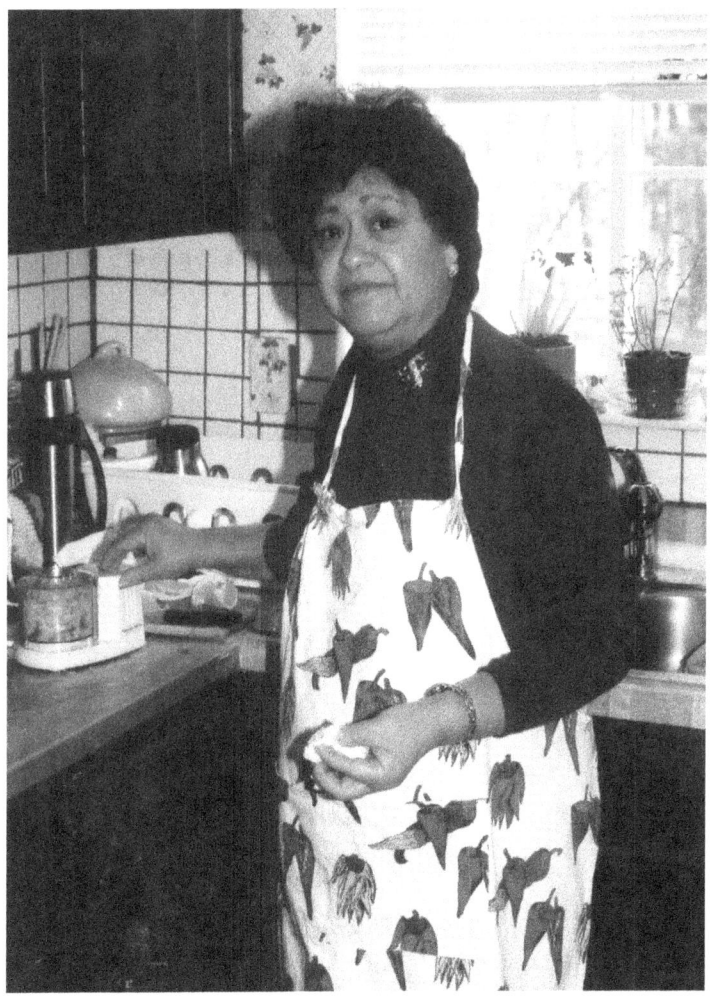

Celia in cooking mode

September 2007—I now spend twenty-four hours per day, seven days per week, providing the most personal and delicate assistance conceivable to another person. My day revolves around such things as the time and type of bowel movements, the weight and color of wet diapers, and the size and shape of a piece of bread.

And then there is the matter of our interpersonal relationship. I no longer enjoy any semblance of respect, love, or affection from my wife of thirty-eight years. She despises me completely. In her mind, I am a combination of her jailer and Nurse Ratchett. (You might recall that Nurse Ratchett cared very sternly for Jack Nicolson's character in One Flew Over the Cuckoo's Nest.) Celia can't eat or drink unless I help her to do so. She cannot get on the toilet, brush her teeth, or take a shower without me laying hands on.

I administer her dreaded medications. There are numerous medications that she thinks do her no good at all. Of course the prescribing doctors say they actually do, but she doesn't realize it. Without her medications, she howls at the top of her lungs that I am a cowardly son of a bitch and a bastard for not killing her as she exhorts me to do every day. With her medications she is just plain angry and nasty toward me (and toward God, for that matter), and the decibel levels are lower.

One of the most energetic, vivacious people you can imagine is fast becoming an invalid with little control over her body, her mind, or her spirit.

Any overlap between reality and Celia's perception thereof became more and more accidental. She could look at two pills lying right in front of her and swear that she had already swallowed them. She would then accuse me of trying to double medicate her by sneaking two more pills in front of her. She had a prescription for Xanax to quell anxiety. She often refused to swallow it, however, because she thought it was part of a plot on the part of her doctor and me to control her.

She started resisting my every verbal direction vehemently. She saw my requests as being bossed around by me. It immediately put her into a rage. The most well-meaning suggestion or physical boost met with her sudden and extreme resistance.

I had to explain to my neighbors that Celia sometimes yelled loudly out of frustration, and that there was no need to summon the police. I was not abusing her, even though it must certainly have sounded that way to the neighbors at times.

The boys were able to travel out from Virginia to join us for Christmas 2007 in Vegas. We also convinced Celia's baby sister, Delia, to join us. She drove in from Santa Cruz, California. She is a single-career high school teacher.

A great time was had by all. We had a large Christmas tree with more gifts than would fit. Scott and Sean took turns racing Celia's electric scooter around the house and the driveway. Delia taught Scott, Sean, and Ellie how to make tamales. They somehow managed to permanently stain our white porcelain kitchen sink red. The last thing on our minds was that it would be our last Christmas together.

Celia ended 2007 permanently in a wheelchair. She briefly underwent some balance therapy that did not help her balance at all. The therapy involved suspending her in a harness that was attached to a track in the ceiling by a bungee cord. The failure of the therapy actually contributed to a final diagnosis of neuropathy that paralyzed both legs and the nerves that controlled bodily functions. We tried a rented electric wheelchair, but her mental acuity was not up to the task of guiding it on her own. Our brand new refrigerator took a real beating because she could not use the joystick steering device in a steady manner. I got her an electric three-wheeled scooter, but her ability to operate it on her own was short-lived. I used it for more than a year as an electric wheelchair around the house. I put her in it, turned her around to face backward, and I drove it backward while walking behind her.

For a few months, she stubbornly tried to walk around the house or stand at the stove in the kitchen and cook. These attempts got her another trip to the emergency room with a cracked rib. Once again, she had to certify to the emergency room nurse that I had not inflicted the injury upon her.

I even got injured once when I caught her before she fell against a coffee table. She ended up fine, but I tore my rotator cuff.

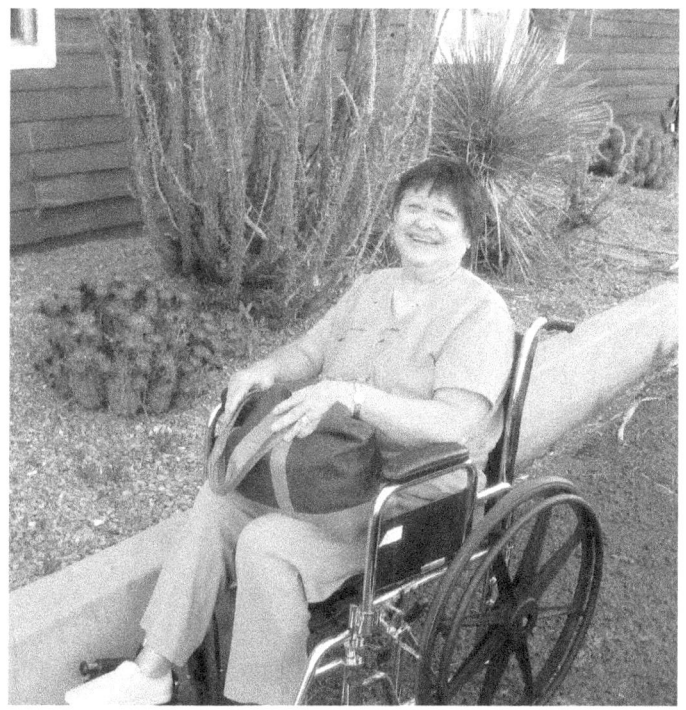

Celia wheeling around Las Cruces, NM, in the summer of 2008

Chapter Three

Caring for the Caregiver—Yourself

February 2008 —*You are a caregiver—not a robot. You have feelings too. Every once in a while you will be forced to react to the shabbiness of the treatment you receive from that person. One of the first things I read during an Internet search about caring for the emotionally infirm was that confrontation is not of any use and is not recommended.*

I learned the truth of that for myself. At first, I would respond to Celia's insults and harangues by hollering back at her that I was just helping her. I did nothing other than to help her. I would tell her over and over the word *help, help, help*. It meant nothing to her. All she knew was that things were not as she wanted them right then and there. All she wanted was for me to change them. Arguing about how things were was the epitome of futile.

My first attempt to deal with my frustrations was very simple. I began by trying the counting-to-ten routine. It helped somewhat. Then I read another Internet article by a holistic healing guru that talked about breath control as a stress reliever. He asserted that if we all just breathed as naturally and deeply as a newborn baby, we would have less stress. It sounded reasonable to me. It also sounded easy to do under any circumstance. I did it for many months and I found it pretty effective. When she got totally unreasonable, I went to another room and took three deep breaths (just three as the guru recommended). I didn't want to hyperventilate.

April 2008 —*She forgets quickly. Her short-term memory loss is actually a benefit in this regard. Twenty minutes after a very vicious, hateful flare-up she calls to me (I am in the other room breathing) to ask if she can have another glass of root beer. She is even-tempered and docile. She is watching CNN Headline News for the twenty-fifth iteration of the same story.*

I came to realize that life's lessons really were continual. Some years ago, in the early eighties, I thought that I had ascended Maslow's hierarchy of human needs to its highest point of "self-actualization." I was in one of my more rewarding army assignments. It was an assignment as the head of a twelve-man teaching/training team based in San Francisco. I was a captain, and my team consisted of two warrant officers and nine senior noncommissioned officers. We were part of a group of teams. Our jobs were to teach/train reserve component units located throughout California and Nevada. We were "regular army" guys (meaning full-time active duty soldiers) who were to impart our knowledge and skills to our US Army Reserve and National Guard counterparts. We tried to help them be more ready to activate and serve along side regular army units in time of war. Ironically, that activation seemed remote and unlikely back in the eighties. It has since become a longstanding reality in Iraq and Afghanistan.

My tough care duties made me realize that self-actualization was not a final destination. Maslow's hierarchy is climbed and re-climbed any number of times over the course of a lifetime. I had regressed to where I had to function at the level of some pretty basic needs, both hers and mine. It was meaningless that I thought I had previously achieved his highest state on a number of occasions during my army career and afterward as a founding partner and leader in a small business. I was reminded every day how basic needs can motivate really base behaviors.

Celia's extremely angry and aggressive behavior sometimes elicited from me purely visceral responses. I never responded physically, but I certainly went toe-to-toe with her in very vehement verbal assaults.

As with anything, practice made perfect. I practiced restraint every hour of every day. The days turned into weeks, months, and then years. I learned not to respond in kind, no matter the provocation.

July 2008 —*The spectrum of her emotions runs the gamut from happy, through sad, to anger and rage. It is seasoned with good measures of fear and paranoia as well. I have attempted to picture what a bell-curve distribution of her moods might look like. I believe it would be skewed heavily toward the anger/rage side of the scale.*

Starting from left to right, I pictured a small area of about ten percent consisting of happiness such as a giggle or laugh at something funny on a Seinfeld rerun or a smile at the picture of our new granddaughter. The next area under the curve would be maybe another 10 or 15 percent of listlessness and general sadness. Then would begin the largest area under the curve. It would be abut 50 or 60 percent anger and bitterness about all things. Although I realized intellectually that this anger was really aimed at her terrible situation, I am the only person around to receive its brunt every day and every night. The last area under the skewed curve would be a small tail of 10 percent verbal rage (at guess who?) and finally physical rage and attack. I had been bitten several times. I had dodged being bitten a number of times. Whenever I attempted to help her with any physical move, I had to literally wrestle with her as she attempted to squirm free of my grasp in order to throw herself to the ground while I tried to assist her to move from a wheelchair into another seat or vice versa. This seat-to-seat transfer, of necessity, had to happen at least six times a day, but more likely eight or ten times. Each transfer was a verbal and physical contest. I always won by dint of my size versus hers, but it really was quite wearing on us both. She did have the advantage of limited short-term memory, however. Within fifteen minutes of the nastiest altercation, she had forgotten it completely. I did not get that luxury.

November 2008 *—Tough care requires a lot of gut checks on the part of the caregiver. Logic and rationality do not apply when caring for a loved one who is no longer capable of loving you, or anyone else. Pure guts and determination carry the day—day in and day out. She alternately loves and hates her own children, her own siblings, everyone around her. It changes hourly and abruptly.*

While I am rendering help to her that is of the most pressing and basic kind, she is viciously assaulting me with insult after insult. I do everything for her that she cannot do for herself. Before, during, and after giving that care, I am lambasted as a liar, a sneak, and someone who is plotting to kill her. I am the most brutal man, and the least caring person she knows. According to her I break both her arms and legs several times per day while helping her into and out of a bed or a chair.

She either begs or demands that I help her die every day. She would prefer death to her current state of handicap, both physical and mental. When she is not exhorting me, she is exhorting God to do the same. I don't know about him, but I simply cannot do it. I now see the truth to the idea that there are no atheists anywhere near death. Any military chaplain will tell you that there are no atheists in battle. You can't take the chance that you will need somewhere for your soul to go any minute. Nonchalance disappears.

I finally accepted the fact that the same sort of thing happens to anyone in close proximity to death, not just on the battlefield, but in the home or the hospital. Nonchalance about what happens after death was no longer a theoretical thing. It was real, tangible, and right in front of me. It had a face. I touched that face constantly. A friend told me that the only way he had overcome his young daughter's sudden death was to believe she was now with God, regardless of my friend's personal beliefs (or disbeliefs) over a period of years. A year before her death he would not have given God a second thought. God became the reason my friend could still get up and go to work in the morning.

Christmas 2008 *—Celia's emotions ebb and flow unpredictably. She has constant ups and downs. In her case, the baseline is now simple anger and spitefulness. It descends into bitterness, hurtfulness, and rage, at the drop of a hat.*

I must live my life on the basis that there is only her, always attending to her needs first. Before I brush my teeth, take my vitamins, get some food, or go to the bathroom, I must first be sure all of those things are done for her. At mealtime, I generally just eat whatever she leaves. This is no big deal, as I have a few extra pounds on me anyway.

Chapter Four

Endurance

February 2009 —*I am confirming my long-held belief that stress is actually external pressure that you internalize—or not. I can either let her extreme behavior penetrate me to the point that it is a stressor or not. I strive every day to succeed at limiting the amount of external pressure I permit to become internal stress. Stress kills, and I will have no more of that. I have had quite enough over these last few years.*

More and more often, I find myself thinking about my ancestors who were Irish coal miners in northeast Pennsylvania. They endured the worst kind of daily drudgery under miserable and dangerous conditions. They did this day in and day out for decades —for their entire lives. I am beginning to know their situation. I face daily drudgery of the physical, mental, and emotional kinds. I use the picture of them toiling in their dark cold pits to chip away at endless mountains of hard coal and rock to lift my spirits. My drudgery seems equally endless and difficult, but at least it takes place in a comfortable home, safely above ground. I have a nice HDTV and the Internet and lots of reading material (courtesy of my new eReader). As a full-blooded Irishman, I am not really prone to experiencing excessive stress. I think the arithmetic of nature combined with nurture applies here. I am, by nature, inclined to not internalize pressure very much. I am also highly inclined, by both nature and nurture, to apply various and sundry alcohol-based elixirs to high-pressure and potentially stressful situations.

This was the case since my early teenage years. In fact, my not-so-illustrious military career actually began when cheap whiskey, fast women, and faster cars all combined to place me in front of a municipal court judge. He warned me that my next choice would be the army in Vietnam or jail. I chose the army. Due to reasons entirely beyond my control, the army sent me to Germany rather than to Vietnam, but that is another story altogether.

While caring for my wife under pretty tough conditions, alcohol was just not an option. As a *tough care-giver*, I had another person's well-being reliant upon my ability to react quickly, coolly, and correctly at a moment's notice twenty-four hours a day, seven days a week. There was no room for sloppy judgment or even dull judgment during a hangover. If Celia vomited while on her back in bed, it could have choked her to death. I had to always be in earshot of her, if not eyeshot. I had to always be ready to do the right thing, immediately. An inexpensive set of baby-monitoring speakers became a necessity.

In March of 2009 we got one of those welcome breaks of good news. Scott and Ellie provided us with our first grandchild. Alexandra Pelagia Mooney was born on 19 March 2009. The last few months of Ellie's pregnancy were very stressful for Celia. She told her sister and her neurologist both that she did not understand why the baby was taking so long to be born. Just before the delivery, she was convinced that Ellie had been pregnant for fourteen months. There was no mathematical or medical opinion that could convince her otherwise.

I found myself managing pressure/averting stress through several means:

The deep breathing exercise I discussed previously is the one I used the most frequently. It required little time and no special materials. It could be done anywhere, anytime.

I engaged in a project to digitize all our accumulated family photographs and upload them to the Internet. This project ended up lasting much longer than I expected. I looked at almost thirteen thousand photographs that started somewhere around 1950 and ended around 2004 or 2005. All of our photos since then were taken with digital cameras, and most of them had already been posted to an Internet photo storage site. It was a very mundane and laborious job to review, sort, and scan that many photos. I ended up sending most of them out to a bulk scanning firm and paid a nickel a picture for about ten thousand. Three thousand photos turned out to be too blurry or completely unidentifiable to bother scanning and processing. In retrospect I did create a very interesting photo history that spans several hemispheres and oceans, several family trees, and lots of friends. It is now available to our future generations. I found hundreds of photos of Celia in happier, more active days. Many of them were taken in our yards and flower gardens in various places where we had lived over the years. The most recent ones showed her at our house in northern Virginia, where she grew countless flowers and many types of hot chili peppers. She epitomized the term *green thumb*.

Celia had grown up in an agricultural family. Her early years were spent on the road with her entire family moving from state to state. They picked whatever was in season, mostly fruits and vegetables. They wandered as far north as Michigan. They did settle for a number of years near Las Vegas and their large extended family there. They also migrated through Arizona and Utah. Their first permanent home was in Fresno, California, where their dad settled in as a farm supervisor until his retirement many years later.

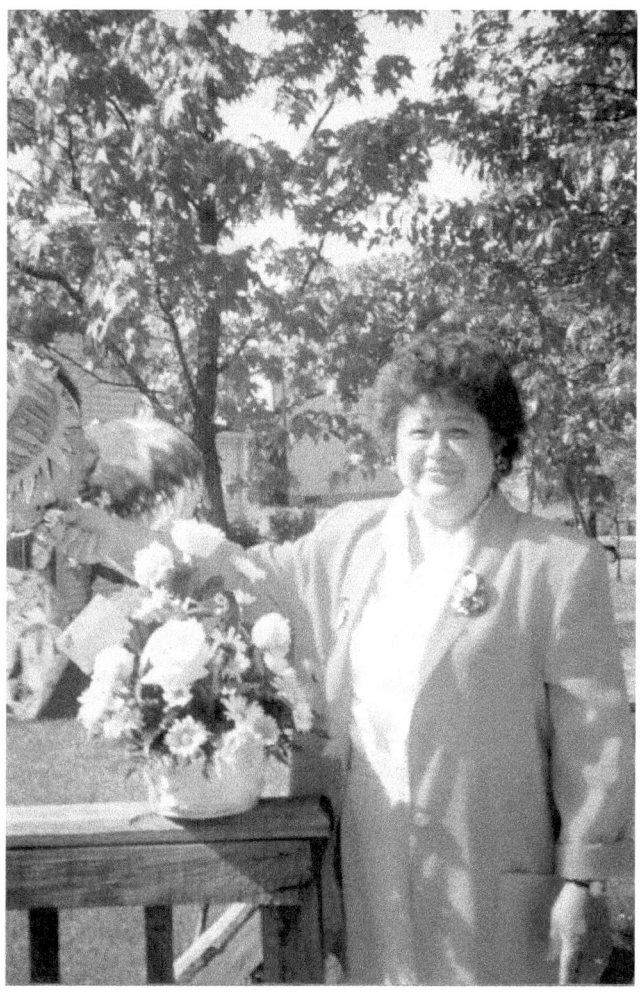

Celia with her ever-present flowers and greenery

I also sought relief by becoming an amateur on-line investor. It accomplished two critical goals —it let me make money (more or less) without leaving the house, and it consumed a pretty good chunk of time in research (or due diligence, as they call it in the investment lingo) and trading. The stock market exercised and stretched my mind. It was enough of a challenge that it was a worthwhile distraction from my other, more mundane, responsibilities. It also ended up paying the bills, since I could not pursue a profession that would take me out of the house or on the road.

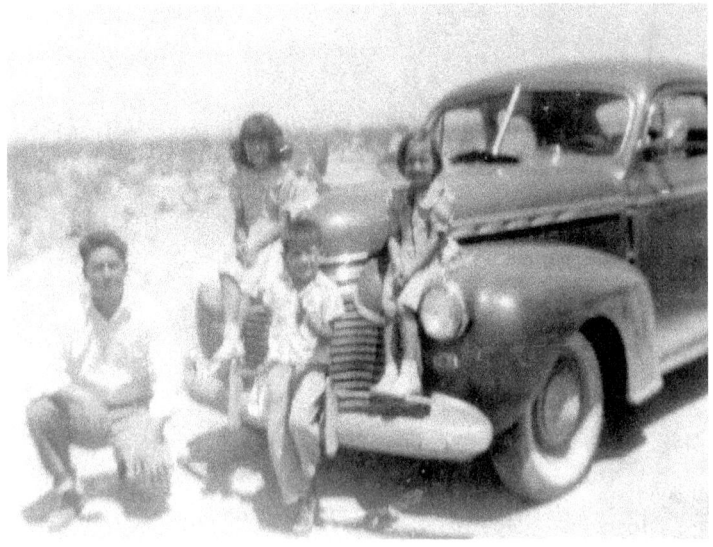

Celia (top, left) traveling through the desert with her family

I spent some hours playing computer mah-jongg. I occasionally alternated it with computer solitaire, but solitaire didn't really tax the mind enough to distract it. I learned how to regularly wipe a mah-jongg board in under two minutes.

I read a great deal. My sons got me an eReader last Christmas. I loved it and read voraciously. WWII history had always interested me because my father served in the army as a grunt (i.e., infantryman) from 1942 to the end of the war. I have read a lot of general WWII history books and some that are specifically about the campaigns my father was involved with in North Africa, Sicily, Italy, France, and Germany. Other reading materials included historical biographies like that of Benjamin Franklin and pure fiction, such as Ayn Rand's *Atlas Shrugged*.

I wrote this quasi-journal about my experiences as a tough caregiver. It really was cathartic to dump these thoughts and feelings down on the screen rather than shout them back at her blank, confused face.

May 2009 —I must always control my response to her worsening behavior. She becomes ever more caustic and contrary. She ignites at the slightest provocation, however well intentioned by me. I must swallow hard and just keep helping her. Ten minutes after a vicious attack against me, she has forgotten that it occurred. I do not forget, however, and it adds to the heap of hurt I accrue every passing day. Again, I am forced to recall my ancestors who labored in the coals mines of Pennsylvania. If they could do that day in and day out for years, then I can endure this.

I continue to follow my gut reaction and refuse her daily exhortations to kill her or help her to kill herself in order to put her out of her misery. Her misery is great. She has always been very independent, energetic, and action oriented. Just sitting still for hours, days, weeks, months, and now years in a row really is the ultimate misery for her. I hope my instinct against assisted suicide proves to be right. I can certainly see her side of things.

Another aspect to a blue-collar, Irish dirt farming ancestry is a decidedly unromantic conception of love. I was caring for a loved one. I was committed to see her through her illness, however long it took and however terrible it was. This commitment stemmed from a love that was never demonstrated in any storybook, romantic way. Our long marriage, like so many others before and since, was based on a much more common form of love that was expressed on a daily basis more by simple action and silent support than by words or gestures. We were never Romeo and Juliet. I noticed this pattern with my parents during their fifty-something years together. I also saw it in Celia's parents, both natives of Mexico.

Recall that in ancient Rome there were two classes of free men—the aristocratic patricians and the common plebeians. I think that most people practice a very plebian love. It is simple and understated (sometimes to the point of unstated). It manifests itself in daily actions of respect and support and affection. It is contrasted against the obvious and flamboyant patrician form of love that I think may exist only in books and on the screen.

By May, the brand new grandma was twitching in her wheelchair to see the baby.

Commercial transportation was out of the question. Her impatience soon went to the point of obsession. She was sure she would "never" see the baby. I loaded up a small utility trailer with some items the boys wanted to get back from us that we had taken from Virginia when we moved. Celia and I hit the road with trailer in tow at about four PM on a Saturday in mid-May. We had planned to leave early Sunday morning as we had done on numerous car trips in the past, but she awoke on Saturday in a near frenzy to get going. We traveled only for an hour or two. We stopped in Kingman, Arizona, at a motel on Interstate 40. We covered the two thousand remaining miles with some difficulty but made it nonetheless. As it turned out, "Handicapped Accommodations" meant different things to different hotel chains. Getting in and out of the car and the hotel/motel rooms certainly gave us both a real workout for the next three days.

We did finally make it and spent most of the summer of 2009 coddling our new granddaughter and partying with the boys like it was 1999.

We also got a chance for a great semi-family reunion during Thanksgiving of 2009. I rented a large house that provided handicapped access near Santa Cruz, California. Celia and I drove out from Las Vegas a little early and spent two nights with her younger sister, Delia, in Watsonville on our way to Santa Cruz. Scott, Ellie, Alexandra, Sean, and Kayli flew out from Virginia. They stayed a few days with

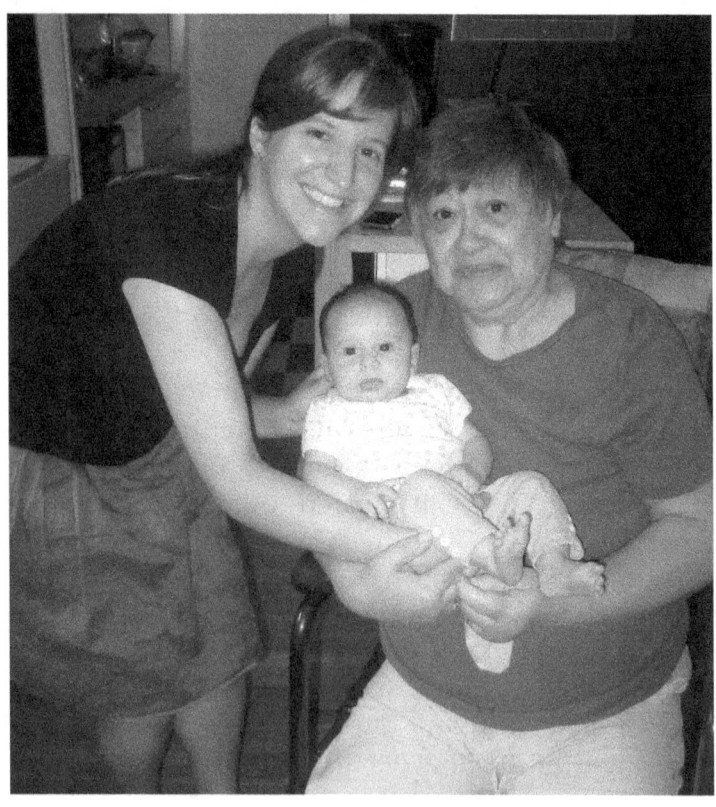

Ellie, Alexandra, and Celia, June 2009

Ellie's brother and sister-in-law, who lived in San Francisco. Delia joined us from nearby Watsonville. We all got together at the large house in Capitola for Thanksgiving dinner. Sean and Delia collaborated on a fine dinner of Turducken and the trimmings. (Turducken is a food made famous by John Madden of NFL fame. It is a turkey stuffed with a duck, which is stuffed with a chicken, which is finally stuffed with Cajun sausage.)

An example of the need for the caregiver to remain mentally alert at all times occurred just after our return from the Thanksgiving gathering in California. In December of 2009, as an exception to the rule, I had left Celia alone for a very short time while I ran out to the nearest fast-food place to grab us some dinner. I left her sitting very securely in a chair placed close to the kitchen table. She was calm and watching one of her favorite cowboy reruns on TV. I told her where I was going and that I would be back shortly. I also left one of the signs I had made up in front of her. It was the one that said, "I am gone to the store. I will be right back."

When I returned after about fifteen or twenty minutes, I found her lying on her stomach on the kitchen floor. The floor was made of hard ceramic tile. At first she did not seem injured. She made no sounds at all. I picked her up and sat her upright in her chair again. I then realized that she had landed fully on her face and forehead.

I immediately rolled her out to the car and rushed her to the nearest emergency room (again).

I got another chance to defend myself from spousal abuse accusations (stated and implied) from the ER nursing staff. Celia did her best to tell them it was another accident. They did CT Scans and X-rays that did not indicate any fractures or breakages. She had one hell of a contusion on her forehead. It generated two black eyes that lasted for over a month.

Control

January 2010 —*I control me. Now I have to also control her. She no longer has any control. No matter how I want to interact with her as a person, I have to realize that I cannot. She functions based on the moment. It is either good or bad right now. It is hot or cold—right now. She is hungry or not. She is tired or not —right now. For her to consider whether she should eat now or wait a little while is like considering whether to launch a mission to Mars or not. They are equally complex problems to her.*

I must retain complete control of my feelings, reactions, and actions. It is very tempting to react to her, but I cannot. She does not comprehend what she says or what she does as it relates to anything other than herself. She has basically descended Maslow's hierarchy of need to its lowest level. She is back at the bottom. The most basic human needs for security and sustenance are all she knows. In truth, she no longer understands it as a hierarchy.

Our sleep is fleeting. For her it just comes or it doesn't. Sometimes it is blocked by "bad dreams" that she cannot or will not elaborate upon. For me, it is another case of my life now centering on her every whim, mood, or condition. When she is cold she just says that. She cannot think about how to deal with it; she just says it over and over until I hear her and take action. It is the same thing if she is too hot, or hungry or thirsty, or if she is wet or dirty. She is not a self-sustaining, thinking, rational adult anymore. She has reverted to a toddler—a toddler with a temper who uses it liberally.

Logistics got interesting. I spent thousands of dollars on pieces of equipment and supplies. Much of it was wasted. I bought special cushion after special cushion for her several wheelchairs. I rented a Hoveround electric wheelchair to see if she could use it. I was glad I did the test rental. She ran it repeatedly into the refrigerator door. My car had a special seat to assist her in and out of the car that cost seven thousand dollars alone. Still there was no financial support from any source for any of these things I did to care for her.

The insults that she hurled at me were many and varied. As outlined previously, I assisted her with the most basic of human bodily functions. While I was doing those things, I was subjected to insult upon insult. She hated the smell of my breath. Every attempt to help her sit when she could not do so on her own caused her to scream at me for my "brutish' ways. She claimed that I broke both of her arms and legs every time I helped her into or out of bed. My chest and shoulder remain riddled with her bite marks. I got bitten almost daily whenever I assisted her into and out of her wheelchair. She bit out of pure animalistic survival instinct. She thought that since she was not in control of her own standing and sitting, I must have been attempting to drop her to her death, several times per day.

I even nursed her through a yeast infection. I will leave the details unstated and defer to the lady readers to enlighten the men. She suddenly started scratching uncontrollably at her crotch. At first I thought it was just another obsessive way of behaving with regard to a minor itch. I noticed that her genitalia were swollen and distended. I recalled her making reference to a yeast infection some years ago. Back then I did not need to concern myself with things like that, so I would pass them off. I did recall that she always ended up dealing with it without having to see a doctor. Now, however, I was the only one who could take any action —whatever it was. I found some generic over-the-counter pills and gave them to her for two days, with little result. I was about to call an OB/GYN office, and I decided to goggle yeast infection so I could talk to the office more intelligently. The first hit on Google was for an over-the-counter product. I read several sites for symptoms and treatments and concluded that this product administered by me would probably handle it. It did. Another example of how one must be prepared to learn something new every day.

I started noticing changes in her that seemed fairly significant on an almost daily basis. To me as a layman, these changes sorted into three categories— physical, mental, and emotional. Her neurologist reminded me that things were neither that simple nor that discrete. He explained that those three things were closely intertwined and combined to produce whatever it is that I observed.

In the category of things that appeared to me to be physical in nature, I saw the following changes over the recent past:

Her right hand and arm were losing strength and dexterity. She could just barely grasp a spoon or fork. (Knives had been too difficult for a long time already.) Of course, when I attempted to help her eat, she got very angry and frustrated. I began serving her foods that were prepared in such a way that she could pick up a morsel and put it in her mouth manually. I slowly realized that this would also pass before too long, and she would have to get accustomed to me feeding her. For instance, I would cut a baked sweet potato into cubes about an inch across. I made small short ribs that she could handle clumsily with one hand. I cut hamburgers in quarters and served her a lot of baked French fries.

She had almost constant lower back pain and occasional neck pain.

She always slouched to one side or another. She could only sit upright with help from me, or a set of pillows.

She could no longer pick up a drink and just consume it. I had to start the process of getting the cup into her grasp and then help her to lift it to her mouth. After a few sips, the weight of the cup lessened, and she could do the rest herself. Getting the cup back out of her grasp was always a challenge as well. Sometimes I would catch her trying to drink without my help by lowering her face and mouth onto the cup and lapping the liquid like a dog. She also tried this with food once in a while.

I noticed that sometimes she said she did not see a plate of food sitting immediately in front of her, or a cup. Not always, but frequently.

At the suggestion of Celia's neurologist, I took her to an optometrist. She actually put forth a creditable effort at bluffing her way through a standard eye exam. However, her attempt was not successful. It soon became apparent that she could not identify the letters of the alphabet, regardless of how near, far, or large. The optometrist changed from alphabetic charts to pictures that were used for children too young to read. This revealed that her visual acuity had worsened significantly over the past eighteen months, since her last exam. It also caused the optometrist to conclude that she was having trouble processing the images her eyes saw. A birthday cake was the first image, and it took her a minute or two to say that. She recognized it at different sizes and distances. A telephone also finally registered. A person's hand and a car never did. She also had cataracts developing, but not to the extent that would explain her poor performance on the eye exam. The optometrist believed she had a blind spot that encompassed one or both of the lower quadrants of her vision (lower left and/or lower right). His exam indicated her eyes and associated nerve connections were all quite normal and functioning correctly. He thought the blind spots were caused by damage to the parts of the brain that processed those specific quadrants of a person's sight picture. The conclusive test for this condition involved a set of hand/eye coordination tasks that she clearly would not comprehend or be able to respond to at all.

I learned another logistical lesson the day of the eye exam. I took her to a second appointment to have a periodic blood sample taken at the order of her internist. Even with the aid of the new electric Turning Assisted Seat in the car, Celia and I both were physically strained by getting her in and out of the car several times in one day (and getting her into and out of the optometrist's exam chair). We never did more than one appointment in a day again. One appointment per week was really more like it.

Chapter Six

The Beginning of the End

June 2010 —*In the category of things that appear to me to be mental in nature, I see the following changes recently:*

She completes about one sentence in ten. She always starts but then gets stymied at the object of the sentence. For instance, she says: "Can I have a _____?"

The blank being something she wants like a food or drink, or some warm socks. When I start to guess what it might be, it frustrates her and makes her angry. Sometimes she finally remembers, but not usually. She also calls my name frequently. It took me a while to figure out that my name could have many meanings. Sometimes "Bernie" simply meant "Come here." But other times "Bernie" could mean "I'm cold," or "I'm hungry," or "I need to be changed." Sometimes I could tell from the look in her eyes that "Bernie" meant "Please help me end this misery." For quite a while, when I go to her from just a short distance away, she had forgotten why she called me.

She has started going into periods of really distant, blank staring. Sometimes it just occurs. Sometimes I instigate it by asking her a simple question. For instance, I will ask her: "Do you want a drink of water?" Her response will be to stare at me as though I were speaking a strange language. She just stares at me. Again, if I try and repeat the question or press the issue at all, she gets very upset and screams at me for "Asking too many questions!"

In the category of things that appear to me to be emotional in nature, I see the following changes:

Anger remains her dominant emotional state. It starts when her eyes open in the morning and it is there when she gets into bed at night. It remains at a moderate level throughout the day. It flares up from anger into a tantrum about two or three times a day. The tantrums are usually comprised of yelling, screaming, cursing, and trying to bite me when I get close to her while moving her or helping her sit straight or such things that she views as terrible bothers.

However, she has started drifting into periods of what I would call listlessness or bewilderment (or both). I see her watching one of her favorite western reruns (Cheyenne; The Virginian) or sitcom reruns (Two and a Half Men; Seinfeld; Becker). Then I notice she is actually zoned out, with her mouth open and her jaw slack. She will be this way for some minutes, and then she will just "return" and start laughing at a joke or warning a cowboy about the Indians coming over the hill.

She became hypersensitive to her environment, especially sound and touch. The sound of a knife and fork bumping each other inside the utensil drawer in the kitchen while she is watching TV in the family room (twenty feet away) would trigger a tantrum. If I did not announce myself before entering any room where she was sitting, a tantrum ensued. The sound of a coffee cup placed on a coffee table would anger her greatly. When I changed her clothing or underwear (which I did several times daily) she reacted to every touch with a scream of pain. Sometimes she screamed in anticipation of pain before I actually touched her at all.

She was completely unreasonable and irrational about every thing. Sorting out what she wanted to eat could take an hour sometimes. Whatever I offered, she did not want. However, she refused to say what she wanted. If I tried to prompt her by asking about various possibilities, she went into a tantrum about how I always harassed and bothered her. I usually walked away for a while. After I had been gone about five minutes, she would yell for me and wanted to know where her food was, and we would start over.

We went through what I now call the "daffy diaper debacle." She seemed to have contracted another yeast infection. I treated her for yeast infection again. That did not resolve the issue, so I got a prescription antibiotic from her urologist. The most visible symptoms persisted. She itched constantly in and around her private parts. I gave her two more iterations of each treatment. I finally took her to her OB/GYN. This was the first time I ever stepped into the OB/GYN examining room with her in thirty-nine years of marriage, including two children. The OB/GYN doctor tested for yeast infection and found none. However, she said Celia appeared to be having an allergic reaction to the adult diapers she was wearing.

Once again we learned that it is the little things in life that can cause some really big problems. A few weeks earlier, I had to change brands of underwear because the brand she had been wearing for several years was discontinued. I switched from Brand A to Brand B. She was allergic to the latex component in Brand B. The latex, not a yeast infection, was the source of all the itching. Unfortunately, Brand A was taken over by Brand B, and reverting back to the "new" Brand A did not help. I tried Brand C. It was better but still itchy. The OB/GYN doctor recommended getting a seamstress to make cotton panties with flaps for removable cotton pads. In the meantime, I placed a clean washcloth between her underpants and her privates every night at bedtime.

This helped. In the end, I found a latex-free Brand D on the Internet. I thanked goodness and Stanford University for the Internet.

August 2010 —*Her latest bizarre activity is a disgusting one. She has all of her bowel movements in her underwear. She has taken to scratching her rear end in her sleep. If there is fecal matter in her pants at the time, she gets the feces on the fingertips of her right hand. This is the only hand that still works at all. The disgusting part comes when she then bites the fingernails of her right hand. These fingernails are full of feces —pretty bad. I now must watch her to make sure that I wake up and clean her fingers if they are dirty. I try to clean up bowel movements as soon as I know about them, but they often occur at night while we are both asleep.*

Chapter Seven

Professional Help with Tough Care

September 2010 *—In point of fact, she is now completely paralyzed, unable to speak more than a few words, and her mental processes are largely frozen. She recently was visited by two aunts, two uncles, and her brother and his wife. Over the course of two days, she recognized and reacted to these close family members a total of less than one hour. She uttered only a few words over the entire weekend. As usual, she utters at me very loudly whenever I do anything that she does not like. Whenever I move her to change her underwear or to put her in bed, she says quite clearly—"you son of a bitch, you bastard." I believe this blast of vitriol stems from* *two sources. First, it is her way of continuing to curse me for not complying with her demands and pleadings over the past year or two that I kill her and put her out of her misery. Second, it really is just a visceral reaction to being disturbed, which is becoming ever more painful for her by the day. If I dig deeply enough, I start to wonder if it relates back to years of me working (and drinking) too much in the more distant past. Only she knows for sure. I am reminded of I. A. Richards' basic theory that "Meanings are not in words, they are in people."*

In late September 2010, we visited Celia's neurologist. For the first time, he clearly identified dementia as a specific ailment of hers. It was a result of a creeping ischemic disease in her brain that was gradually damaging different regions of her brain that controlled various functions. Her dementia sat on top of earlier stroke aftereffects and neuropathy. He said, "Her brain is approximately twenty or twenty-five years older than her body right now and getting older rapidly."

I asked him quite plainly and directly how it could be the case that among the three medical insurances she and I have paid into for almost forty years, there could not be any form of professional medical assistance to care for her in her current state. He said that as a specialist, it was not within his purview to know about or arrange for any kind of basic daily care. He recommended I take the matter up with her internist. Celia was due for a periodic appointment with the internist anyway, so I took her for a routine blood panel test and then arranged an appointment for one week later.

We saw her internist in the first week of October 2010. His first reaction at the appointment was to praise her unstintingly about how well her blood panel results looked. Her blood sugar, cholesterol, triglycerides, blood pressure, etc. were quite well in line, compared to just five months earlier. These statistical results were a dramatic, positive departure from her past three years of results. He suggested that her sugar control medication could possibly even be stopped. He awaited her response to his praise, but instead got the blankest stare from her that you could imagine.

I interjected myself and explained that she would not be able to answer him because she did not comprehend anything he said and that she was almost completely unable to speak. He then noticed the elephant in the room. I repeated my observation to him that there must be a better, more professional way to care for her than me waking up each day and confronting some new form of illness, injury, or behavior and trying to guess what to do. My commonsense approach to helping her as best I could was no longer sufficient, I told him. I asked what he might be able to do to bring professional medical help to her and me both.

He issued an order that day to a home nursing firm. As the name implies, they provided nursing care to those in need. It is provided entirely at home. An intake nurse visited within a few days. She assessed Celia's basic needs and started a process of visits to our home by a number of registered nurses, nursing assistants, and specialists. I mean a *number* of them. Within seven days of the assessment, six people came to do further assessments or render some sort of care, or both. Once all was said and done, we had eight caregivers, plus the twice-weekly respite care I continued over the last two years. The home nursing was the first assistance we received that was covered by health insurance because of the doctor's order, but respite care remained our sole responsibility in terms of payment. Respite care was basically babysitting of Celia while I ran out and did grocery shopping, my own medical appointments, and the other mundane household tasks that I used to take for granted. The tasks had to be carefully planned and organized to fit into two four-hour periods per week (at twenty-two dollars / hour). I could be away from her only for eight of the 168 hours in a week for any reason.

October 2010 *—We did our semiweekly Internet-based computer conference with Scott, Ellie, and baby Alexandra yesterday. Celia could not wave back at Alexandra or say anything other than a sort of weak "Hi."*

Soon after this, Scott and I decided that we needed to get her back to Arlington to spend time with the boys and Alexandra. We realized that we probably had less than a year left with her. She had last seen Scott, Ellie, and Alexandra in person when they visited us in Las

Vegas in January 2010. Sean and Kayli also flew out and visited in March 2010.

Celia's lack of responsiveness during the video conference caused Scott and me to develop a grand plan. Being Full Blooded Irish (the other FBI) I was born with an innate distrust of grand plans—and I had a bad feeling about this one. However, I did my due diligence on an effort to get Celia back East to spend time with her boys and her granddaughter. The objective of the plan was to transport her back to their home in Virginia on 18 December 2010. This was oriented on the fact that our daughter-in-law's condo would come open at the end of October. I would pay for some modifications to the bathroom, and it would be ready to support Celia and me in early December.

I inquired about one-way air ambulance flights. The least expensive was twenty-six thousand dollars. In the end I reserved a large RV one-way for a couple thousand dollars. Scott, Sean, and Kayli would fly out and we would all drive her back, with her in bed the whole way. Kayli was a third-year nursing student. I would order a hospital bed for delivery there in Virginia.

Celia's home nursing case manager was an experienced RN. On her very first visit, on October 12, she examined and treated Celia for some minor bedsores. At the end of her visit, she told me that she was quite certain that home nursing care was not really the appropriate treatment for Celia. She explained that she saw all of the indications that Celia should immediately start receiving some sort of hospice care instead. She explained that she judged Celia's remaining life span to be fewer than six months.

It struck me like a ton of bricks that this visiting nurse was the first medical person in several years to introduce the concept that Celia's condition was terminal, finite, and actually very limited. The case manager believed that Celia met both of the Medicare criteria for hospice care—1) fewer than six months to live and 2) deterioration of mental and physical capacities beyond the point of standard nursing care.

Although it shook me, this information was in line with the gut feeling that I had been harboring for some time. Her condition had been worsening at an accelerating rate for about two months, since late August 2010. Her case manager believed that this was a sign that Celia had undergone a sort of "stealth stroke." It might have been an actual stroke suffered in the dead of night and not noticed by me. Alternatively, it might have been the accumulated effects of numerous TIAs. TIA's are Transient Ischemic Attacks. They are very small disruptions of the tiny blood vessels that carry oxygen throughout the brain. In either event the net effects can be the same. In Celia's case, it was loss of the use of the right arm and loss of speech (both of these controlled on the left side of the brain).

Between 12 and 26 October, Celia and I saw eight home nursing folks. I had to put together a roster to keep them straight. I had all of their contact numbers and used the numbers to coordinate their visits. They were all consummate professionals. All of the therapists stopped by one time, each for a few minutes, and quickly determined that there really was nothing more they could do. The nurses and Certified Nurse Assistants (CNAs) came regularly and treated her bedsores and helped me bathe her.

The case manager/RN formalized her recommendation for a change to hospice care to Celia's internist. He ordered that a home hospice assessment be done.

Chapter Eight

The End State

On October 28, 2010, an experienced and specially trained hospice RN visited to perform an assessment of Celia's condition. After about fifteen minutes, she concurred that hospice care was most certainly in order. She offered me the choice of inpatient or home hospice care. I decided on the home option. Celia was categorized as suffering from end-stage CVA. The term *CVA* is an acronym for cerebrovascular accident. The term *end stage* was self-explanatory. All hospice care would be paid for by Celia's Medicare entitlement. We discussed the matter of moving her to Virginia. The nurse agreed that it might be feasible if we chose to do it.

Celia's remaining time with us was once again was left unclear. My hesitant but persistent queries generated reminders that hospice care nurses were "not God." Increments of time dwindled rapidly from months, to weeks. In actuality it turned out to be just days.

The hospice concept is based on palliative care. It attempts to provide medical care and services to improve the quality of life for the patient and family. The word *hospice* literally means "a place of shelter." Home-hospice care provides extensive services to terminally ill patients. Care usually involves relieving symptoms, minimizing pain, and providing psychological and social support. The hospice philosophy provides for the spiritual and cultural needs of the patient and family. The goal of hospice care is to provide the terminally ill patient peace, comfort, and dignity.

Hospice care at home helps a family as a whole. Right in the comfort of the home, family members can take an active role in providing all sorts of care and comfort to the patient. Hospice services include a diverse team to help deliver care, including physicians, nurses, social workers, chaplains, home care aids, trained volunteers, pharmacists, and bereavement counselors.

The palliative care relieved Celia's symptoms of pain, shortness of breath, fatigue, constipation, nausea, loss of appetite, and difficulty sleeping that she had been experiencing more and more with each passing day. It helped her gain the strength to carry on with daily life. It improved her ability to tolerate medical treatments. It also helped me have more control over her care by better understanding her overall treatments.

The point of palliative care was to relieve suffering and provide the best possible quality of life for both the patient and their family. It certainly achieved those objectives in our case.

I started another roster of visiting players. As with the home nursing crew, the home hospice staff consisted of a team of very competent and professional RNs, CNAs, and specialists. In our case most of the specialists were rather redundant. Nutrition, occupational, and speech therapists all had very little to do. Since the last visit to Celia's internist in early October, I had not spoken to an MD. I was briefly bothered by that, but then I realized that nurses are the backbone of this type of care. No amount of bedside manner or professional certifications was going to change the direction of this train.

A social worker came by and we reviewed all the legal documents and other administrative arrangements that one needs to have in place during this time. I had previously helped my mother through the illness and passing of my father. Therefore, I had already done the three basic documents pertaining to Celia. I had long ago executed a last will and testament; a medical directive; and a general, durable power of attorney. Additionally, the hospice agreement required the execution of a DNR, or Do Not Resuscitate, order. This permitted any emergency care personnel to refrain from reviving her. None of the hospice staff would do so, by definition. In fact, the hospice agreement included a restriction against calling 911. Any use of medical assistance to prolong her life was a violation of the hospice agreement and would curtail that hospice care altogether.

Celia's home hospice case manager was also an experienced RN. She quickly set up a completely new set of medicines that dispensed with pretty much everything that had been previously prescribed. Neither Aricept nor Lexapro had been doing her much good for some time, apparently. All new meds would be administered by me in the form of liquids in an eye-dropper. The two principal meds were methadone and morphine (immediate release). These were powerful pain medications. The hospice nurse/case manager explained the concept of palliative care, wherein the patient is dealt with entirely on the basis of minimizing pain and suffering while they die.

On November 4 I told her hospice nurse/case manager about the family's grand plan to get Celia back east. She listened quietly, and then suggested that we sit down and talk. She tactfully but firmly made me realize that the three of us were now involved with the natural culmination of Celia's life. She explained that Celia's time remaining was measured in weeks, not months. Moving her to the east coast on 18 December was really not in the cards. In fact, moving her anywhere other than a local hospice facility was not advisable.

I conveyed this new information to Scott, and we decided that it was time for Plan B, as we used to say in the army. I scrubbed the grand plan to make the big RV road trip. The boys, Ellie, and Alexandra would come out to Vegas the weekend before Thanksgiving, arriving on 18 November.

November 2010—*It is early in the morning of 5 November. I am up to write because I was laying awake in bed as something kept ringing in my brain while I listened to what might be her last breaths, minute by minute. I told God that I deserved nothing, but I hoped he would grant her the time and ability to see her boys one last time before she goes. They are now due in to see her in less than two weeks.*

A four-decade-long marriage is comprised of deep love and deep hate, and every shade of the emotional spectrum in between. In the end it all comes down to *caring*, no matter how *tough* it is to do.

Chapter Nine

Respect from la Familia

Celia's sudden departure on 9 November really left me with only two regrets:

1) Her sons and her granddaughter did not make it to see her in time, and
2) Her last words to me were both angry and hurtful (deserved or not)

Our younger son Sean was actually boarding an airplane in Washington, DC, to come and see her that very morning, as she was being taken from our home by the funeral parlor. He and his older brother, Scott, had discussed the scheduled trip by all of them to see her on 18 November, and Sean ended up with a deep feeling that he should not wait until then.

Sean learned from me of her passing in the parking lot of McCarran Airport in Las Vegas at about noon on that same day.

When we reached the house, he asked me exactly where she had died. I showed him the hospital bed in our bedroom. He spent a long time in there alone with his mom's fresh memory. I later consoled him as best I could with a phrase that ended up as our mantra for the next few days: "It is okay to cry when your mom dies."

I had phoned Scott with the news of his mom's death while Sean was flying west. The time difference between Vegas and Arlington Virginia is three hours. Early for me was later for the boys. Scott was certainly prepared to hear it. He quickly got himself a ticket on a flight later that day. Arranging a sudden departure for Ellie, Kayli, and baby Alexandra would be very problematic and difficult on them. So the ladies stayed behind and kept the home fires burning while the Mooney Men took proper care of Mom. By 8:00 PM on the day of her death, we three were together in Las Vegas and ready to start a *tough* couple of days.

The boys and I bonded immediately into one cohesive unit. We were really just doing what came naturally to us. We had often gone on what we used to call "Adventure Training" together. Adventure training consisted of trips that the three of us would take once or twice a year from the time the boys were able to travel. Mom was never really the adventurous or outdoor type, so she would not go along. She always found something domestic she needed to do. The boys and I rafted the New River in West Virginia. We snorkeled around Key West, the Bahamas, and Puerto Rico. We went deep-sea fishing, motorcycle riding, and four-wheeling around an old island in North Carolina that Blackbeard the pirate once frequented. We did take Mom along on our overseas adventures. We all went to Europe a couple of times and to Mexico once. She wasn't missing out on those.

The photos at the back of this book cover shows us gathered at the Hofbrau Haus in Munich on Christmas Eve 2000. It was the only place we could find that was open for supper that night.

After informing Scott of his mother's passing on November 9, I had to make several other very difficult calls. The first was to her brother Ramiro. Fortunately, he had been over to our place to visit with his sister just a few weeks earlier. He had been one of the few people who penetrated her mental and emotional haze and gotten her to laugh, smile, and cry on that visit. He took the news very hard, as expected. Ramiro was the surviving man of the Mendez family. Their parents had both passed some years ago. I next called the youngest of the Mendez clan—Delia. She had last seen her older sister in November 2009 at the Thanksgiving gathering near Santa Cruz, California. She was devastated also. She ended up driving from Santa Cruz to Las Vegas with friends because the drive would have been too much for her to undertake alone. I last called to notify the middle sister, Belia. I had to make this call circuitously through an aunt and through Belia's husband, Speedy. Belia needed to be with someone when she heard the news to ensure that her own poor health did not strike her down as well. I finally got the right communication channel established and let her know what she did not want to hear. She became quite the trooper in response to her sister's passing. She took over the whole matter of gathering the large extended family and keeping them fed for several days. As the sibling who lived nearest, Belia had regular contact with us over the past four years. In fact, she brought a beautician to our home on the day before Celia passed. We were getting her ready for the planned visit by the boys later in November.

The boys and I now faced Mom's passing and the intense family gatherings together—seamlessly. I never once wondered what Scott or Sean might be discussing with a distant relative that they probably did not recognize at all. I knew instinctively that they were being mature, polite, and supportive. They did their mom proud in every way over those days.

I, myself, was on autopilot. The necessary had to be dealt with first, then the important, then the mundane. Fortunately I had the two best wingmen a dad could want.

On Thursday, November 11, Belia put together a family gathering of Celia's extended family at our house. Her brother, sisters, uncles, aunts, cousins, nieces, nephews, great uncles, and great aunts gathered with Scott, Sean, and me. They came from several states. We welcomed each and every one. Some of them we greeted in their native Spanish. Language diversity has always been valued in our home and always will be. Why would anyone ever allow a simple thing like language to stand in the way of communication at a time like this? I am sure Celia was listening intently—and correcting my poor pronunciation of her family's native tongue, as usual.

On Friday, November 12, in a Memorial Chapel in Las Vegas, we held a memorial service for her. The priest who presided over it told me that it was one of the largest groups at a memorial service he had ever addressed in a number of years of performing this function in Las Vegas. The sign-in register contained sixty-four entries, and I believe there were at least another dozen who did not get around to signing the register. I was asked to make a few remembrances to the collected family members who were there. This is basically what I said to them:

"Good evening. As most of you know, I am not noted for long-winded speeches, so rest assured that my words here will be brief. The first two words that occur to me, however, are *thank you*. On behalf of Scott, Sean, Ellie, Alexandra, Kayli, and myself I thank you for coming here to pay your respects to Celia this evening. I know that many of you made trips that were both difficult and expensive to come here from distant places. We thank you very much.

As I look across this gathering of Mendez's, Longorias, Villarreal's, and others, it is clear to me that I don't have to explain to you that life is not always a bowl of cherries. Let me assure you that Celia's life over the past several years has been about as far from a bowl of cherries as one can get. She suffered greatly. But now, as the good padre has explained to us, she is in a different place. She is in a better place where life actually is pretty much a bowl of cherries and it is that way forever. So once again we thank you for coming here and joining us in paying our respects tonight."

On Saturday morning, November 13, I faxed a request for burial in Arlington Cemetery to the Funeral Services Division there. It included a copy of Celia's DD 214, which documented her honorable discharge from the US Army in 1972 after eight years of active service. I also sent the following notice (via e-mail and /or printed note) to our far-flung set of friends from our military and professional careers.

"Dear friends,

It is my sad duty to report that Celia has passed on. A stroke took her quietly and peacefully in the early morning hours on 9 November here at home in Las Vegas.

As many of you know, she had a major stroke in September 2005. It appeared at first that she would not have any major effects. But starting in June 2006 (just after Scott and Ellie's wedding in Crete) her mental faculties became impaired and she lost the use of her left arm and hand. Then diabetes caused severe nerve damage in her lower extremities.

She and I retired to Vegas in late 2006. By late 2007 she was wheelchair-bound and remained so. We traveled back to Virginia in the summer of 2009 to see Scott and Ellie's lovely daughter, Alexandra, who was born that March. Sean lives with Scott, Ellie, and Alexandra in a hundred-year-old home they renovated in Arlington.

Celia's health deteriorated continually through August 2010, when she had another stroke that paralyzed her right arm and hand and left her unable to speak. She entered home hospice care in late October 2010. She was able to say goodbye only to some of her siblings. The boys are currently en route here.

As per her ardent wishes, she will be inurned at Arlington National Cemetery in honor of her proud service in the Women's Army Corps (WAC) and within five minutes of the other sources of pride in her life—Scott, his fine family, and Sean.

Please remember her in your prayers and take care of your health and that of your families."

By 2:30 PM that same Saturday, Scott, Sean, Celia, and I started our last cross- country car trip together from Las Vegas to Virginia. We had made many such trips together over the years on army transfers or on family vacations. This was the ninth or tenth cross-country trip the four of us made together, I think.

It was the first trip of many on which Celia did not complain one single time.

We passed out of Nevada into Arizona over the brand new Hoover Dam bypass bridge. I reflected back on the first time I had traveled the other way, into Las Vegas for the first time. It was in late 1973. I drove a 1973 Pinto wagon carrying myself; Celia; Scott (as an infant); and my younger brother, Mark. It was my first trip west of Pennsylvania. It was also the beginning of many such trips into the southwest for us and our family.

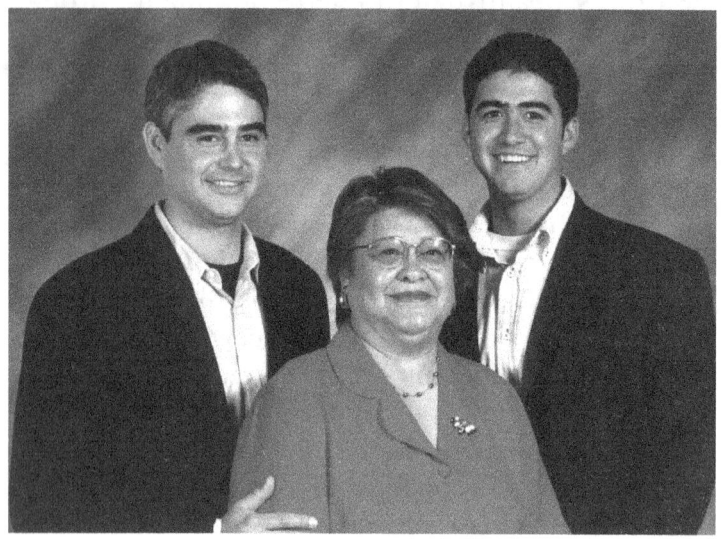

Scott, Celia, and Sean

Chapter Ten

Taps

It took Arlington National Cemetery seven months to finally open its gates to Celia. Once she got on their dance card, however, they handled her funeral service superbly and immaculately. On June 28, 2011, we interred her cremated remains in the Columbarium in the northeast corner of the 624-acre expanse of hallowed ground that has been accepting our nation's fallen since 1864.

We were provided a very nice, private family room to collect ourselves and the family and friends who were joining us that day. It turned out to be myself, Scott, Ellie, Alexandra, Sean, and Kayli, by way of immediate family. Another dozen or so friends who served with us elsewhere in the military and now reside in northern Virginia, and some old neighbors we first met in northern Virginia in 1985, also joined us. Several of Scott's college buddies were there. Several of Sean's high school friends were there as well. Sean's coworkers from his restaurant in Clarendon also joined us. Ellie's mom and two of her brothers were also in attendance. It was an assembly of about twenty-five folks.

We were greeted very respectfully and congenially. We all assembled in a family grieving room, and I completed a few signatures on official documents for the funeral director. He then led us in a vehicle procession about a quarter of a mile to the Columbarium, where her cremated remains would be placed in one of thousands of niches. She is now in a ceramic urn that was made by Scott. Pottery is a hobby of his, but the quality of his work is clearly professional. Ellie sealed the lid on the urn with gold wire.

It was oppressively hot and humid (as only Washington DC, can do hot and humid) at ten o'clock in the morning. Temperature and humidity were both over ninety. Celia's remains and the ceremonial US flag were handled by a seven-man honor guard detachment headed by an army staff sergeant. The leader of the detachment wore the same E-6 stripes as Celia wore when she left the army in 1972. The honor guard placed her remains on a small stand. They then unfolded the ceremonial flag to its full extent horizontally over her remains for just a few minutes. They refolded the ceremonial flag into its well-known triangular shape with only the blue-and-white field of stars showing. The honor guard respectfully handed the flag off to the chaplain who was presiding over the funeral services. At this time a twenty-one-rifle-shot salute was fired in her honor. The twenty-one shots came from seven riflemen who each fired three volleys, or three rounds. They stood at a distance out in the glaring sun. At the end of the twenty-one-gun salute came a playing of "Taps" by a lone bugler off to the left of the ceremonial enclosure. The music echoed off of the marble walls of the columbarium's eight courts that surrounded us. I was reminded of a number of times I had stood at the position of attention in the hot New Mexico sun while assigned to White Sands Missile Range back in the late seventies.

After the military honors were completed, the chaplain led us to the actual niche where her remains will rest forever more. I had planned to carry her urn there myself at this point, but I had not planned for the fact that I would now be in possession of the folded flag handed to me by the chaplain. I tapped Sean on the leg and said, "Go ahead, son. You carry your mother to her final rest." He did so very carefully, erectly, and with great love and care. The chaplain said a few more prayers at the open niche and then Sean placed her in into the niche. Sean, Scott, and I then each placed a memento into the niche along with the urn. I placed the rosary beads that were her favorite because they were personally blessed by Pope John Paul II in a public audience that we attended in Rome in May of 2003. Scott placed a crucifix that was presented to us by the Catholic chaplain who presided over the initial funeral service for Celia in Las Vegas in November. Sean then placed a wooden spoon into the niche with her. The wooden spoon could signify he felt that he had acquired the skills and knowledge and motivation to be a professional chef from his mother, who was a fine cook. But it did not. It signified the principal tool of discipline she used on both of the boys during their formative years.

The entire ceremony described above occurred in a matter of twenty or thirty minutes.

In light of the already oppressive heat, I decided that any words I needed to share with the assembled folks needed to be short and to the point. I made sure everyone knew how much Scott, Sean, Kayli, Alexandra, Ellie, and I appreciated the great efforts they had taken to break away from busy and hectic schedules to come and pay proper respect to their friend Celia as she was laid to rest with the full military honors that she deserved. I told them that I did vaguely recall what it was like to have a busy and hectic schedule, even though it had been quite a while for me. I also invited each of them to join us for an early lunch at a nearby restaurant, which nearly all of them did.

Celia is now finally in the most appropriate resting place possible. It is a place of great honor and great respect. I know that it is absolutely the correct place for her to *rest in peace.*

As it happens, the one-bedroom condo where I live in Arlington is on the edge of Arlington Cemetery. I hear the same "Taps" that are played for her and her new bunk mates every night at eleven PM sharp, just outside my bedroom window.

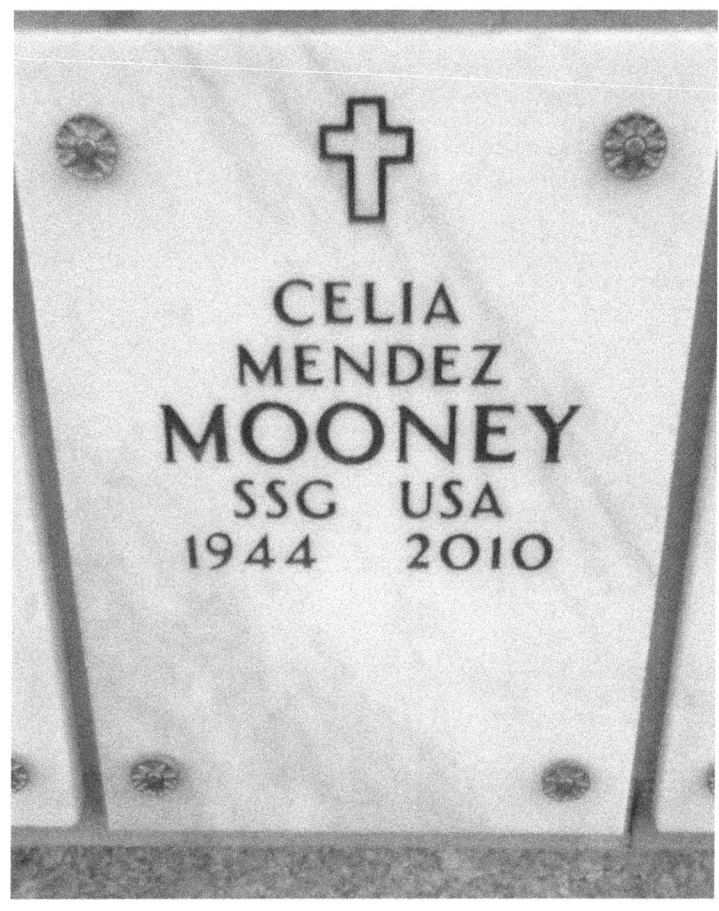

Arlington National Cemetery, Columbarium Court 8

Chapter Eleven

Lessons Learned

I will summarize the main lessons I have learned over the past few difficult years. I hope that these lessons will benefit you (now or in the future). I share these lessons because I believe it is certain that life is too short to learn through your own experience alone. We all need to learn from the experiences of others as much as we can. As I look back on them now, I realize the lessons subdivide into things I learned while caring for Celia under the tough circumstances we had to deal with and lessons about how to handle the passing of your loved one.

During the several years of her care, I learned the following lessons:

The hands of time.

There will be many occasions when you will want to halt and reverse the movement of time. As you watch a bright, strong, energetic person make the slow, steady slide of physical, mental, and emotional deterioration, you will curse the hands of time. Hour by hour, day by day, and year by year, you will have to fight your own depression as you try and minimize your loved one's discomfort and pain. But you cannot change time. You cannot stop it. You cannot reverse it. You must survive it.

You must also be skeptical of all estimates about the time that is left in a person's life. People who are at the end of their lives choose their own time. At some point they realize that it is the end game. I saw Celia resolve within herself that it was time to go. I told her that her boys were coming in just a few days, along with her granddaughter. Celia's baby sister was coming at the same time. She just looked at me with sad eyes and said nothing. For the next several days she refused all food and drink. I am convinced that she took control and left before the people she held most dear could see her in her deteriorated state.

I had to restrain myself from force-feeding her. I put small amounts of water in her mouth with an eyedropper to keep her from being parched. I remembered that the hospice case management nurse explained to me that at this stage, family members often torture the dying person by forcing food and drink on them when it is not wanted, and the frail body cannot process it. The body shuts itself down in an orderly manner. It stops the processing of fuels as it conserves the last bodily energy for the heart and the brain until those lights also go out for the last time.

Perseverence.

Believe me when I tell you that I had many occasions when I wanted to just quit and run away from the situation. Picture yourself supporting the weight of a 135-pound adult with one arm while changing their soiled adult diaper with the other. All the while they scream and holler at you and try and bite chunks out of your chest.

Quitting and running away just is not in the cards, however. They need you, whether or not they realize it. You do realize it. You must do what is right for them just as a parent does for a small child. I was often struck by the full cycle of birth, growth, life, and then death. The end has many similarities to the beginning.

You will be compelled by your own sense of duty and responsibility to soldier on through what will seem to be an endless series of difficulties.

Arguing with someone suffering the effects of dementia (of any form) is absolutely futile. Confrontation does not work. You will be arguing with someone whose mind is no longer capable of rational thought. You will need to endure and continue to care for them, no matter how *tough* it gets.

The simple Serenity Prayer that has long been used in long-term addiction programs came to my mind on a number of occasions.

God, grant me the serenity to accept the things I cannot change,

Courage to change the things I can,

And the wisdom to know the difference.

—Reinhold Niebuhr

Communicate with Doctors.

I really blew this one. I am of the generation that was raised to see medical doctors as all-knowing and always correct. To question a doctor on any medical matter would be anathema to Celia or me. I never have (until recently) questioned anything any doctor said to me. During my *tough care* period, I sat with doctors and with Celia on what may well be a hundred occasions. All the doctors said things that neither she nor I fully understood. Beginning in June 2006, after the parking lot "fender bender" in her internist's office, I began accompanying her to all medical appointments. It became immediately evident that she no longer understood anything that she was being told. I understood better, but still not as fully as I should have.

Doctors are carrying huge patient loads, and they are forced to practice medicine these days in a very litigious environment. Every word they say and action they take exposes them to legal attack. Consequently, they tend to communicate in a rather guarded way. Internists have a tendency to narrowly focus on statistics. They get blood panels done on a patient and then prescribe medications and/or remedial actions on the part of the patient. Some time passes, and then another blood panel and the resulting statistics fall within prescribed parameters—or they don't. Another cycle of medications and/or patient actions ensues. I saw this cycle repeated countless times for Celia (and myself) over the past few years. All the while she was losing mental, physical, and emotional abilities at a rapid pace. At the end, her blood panels were looking spiffy, though.

Specialists limit themselves to their specialties. You should question anything that any doctor says that you do not fully understand. As an example, dementia has more than one form. Which form are you dealing with? How is it best dealt with? Blood sugar can change very abruptly with weight loss, irrespective of medications. Ischemic disease described on a radiologist's interpretive report does not really inform the casual reader very fully about the prognosis or time frame associated with it.

Nurses.

Nurses are the backbone of medical care. I hold them in great respect.

In the military services, the first thing a young officer learns is that the Noncommissioned officers (NCOs) are the backbone of military leadership. This has been proven over centuries. Commissioned officers may be the more educated and cultured leaders, but the NCOs actually get things done. The NCOs get face to face with the troops and cause the soldiers to execute their duties according to their training.

TOUGH CARE

The same is true of nurses in relation to physicians. It was a nurse who first informed me that Celia
was fast approaching death. It was nurses who then
cared for her every day until the day she died. Nurses
visited us every day, sometimes several times per day.
A nurse judged what medication(s) would best provide the palliative care Celia so desperately needed.
The nurses occasionally consulted with a physician
via phone to keep the dispensing of powerful narcotics in compliance with the law. Not once did I see a
physician question or override any nurse's judgment.
Whether it was intentional or not, all of Celia's nurses
and nurse's aides were female. They all used better
bedside manner than I ever saw from any physician
of any gender. A person's end needs to be a gently
respectful time. The nurses who cared for Celia from
the first day of home nursing through to the morning of her death were gentle, kind, and caring. They
could see her silent pain much better than I could.
They told me what to do to alleviate it and I did exactly as they said.

Help is necessary—get it.

I learned this lesson too late. As a man caring for
a woman, I felt physically, mentally, and emotionally
strong enough to care for her. I would like to think
that I did a creditable job. But it is now clear to me,
looking back, that I should have tried harder to get
her better, more professional help sooner. The key to
that help is an order from a doctor to another health-
care provider. Absent that written order, you are on

your own—in terms of physical help and/or financial help. I paid for respite care (aka babysitting) for her for most of two years without any reimbursement or coverage.

Hospice.

It is the most humane way to help your loved one to pass. Whether it is done in an institution or at home, it is a good thing. As a healthy man caring for a slight, frail woman, the choice of home hospice was easy for me to make. It might not be the way to go for a frail healthy older woman caring for a large ailing man. When Celia entered home hospice care she weighed less than a hundred pounds. During the preceding four years she generally weighed around 130 pounds. I still lifted and carried her any number of times per day.

The home hospice environment represented an easing of the physical burden on me. It also lessened the mental and emotional burdens. I now had some medical professionals, rather than just me, who were diagnosing, prescribing for, and caring for my wife. I no longer had to hit the Internet every morning to learn the ins and outs of some new condition or ailment. It was clear to me that Celia also became more calm and comfortable with the kind, gentle nurses' hands—rather than my clumsy mitts—treating her and bathing her.

After her passing, I learned the following lessons, thus far:

Guilt.

You will feel guilt whether or not you deserve to be guilty. You will feel the universal survivor's guilt because you are still alive and your mate is not. The two of you have shared every good thing and every bad thing for a very long time. You faced it all together. Now you feel guilty that she no longer has the opportunity to experience the things that are still to come. These feelings of guilt are unavoidable. You know she will not see any more of her children's successes. She will not be there to watch her granddaughter write the alphabet for the first time.

The trick is to not let this guilt turn into blame. You did not end her life. Her life ended due to circumstances beyond her control and yours, whatever those circumstances were.

You will also feel some more personalized guilt about things that only you and she knew. These are matters that can be settled only by you over the fullness of time. Remember, you cannot reverse time. You will have to thrash these matters out, relying on the idea that you did the best you could with what you had—at the time.

Communication Continues.

You should feel free to continue to communicate with your loved one even after they have gone. It will probably be you communicating with yourself about what transpired over the decades you were together. But that doesn't matter. Communication is communication. Face your thoughts and feelings directly and straightforwardly with your loved one. Avoiding direct, honest talk will be just as harmful now as it was when you were both alive.

Memories.

A thirty-nine-year-long relationship generates a lot of memories. In our case those memories spanned a great deal of geography in addition to time. We traveled a great deal. Sometimes it was due to military transfers, and sometimes it was vacation travel that we undertook to be sure our sons grew up knowing the world rather than just their neighborhood. We swam in most of the world's oceans. We were in the Alps, the Andes, the Pyrenees, and the Rockies. We traversed pretty much all the fifty states.

I find myself dealing with my memories the same way my two-year-old granddaughter handles her toys. She has a toy room where her toys stay most of the time. When the mood strikes her, she grabs an armful of toys and drags them out to the living room or kitchen or hallway to focus her attention on them. Someday she will learn to put them back in the toy room, but not yet.

I have established a large memory room in my mind. The memories stay there most of the time. At odd and random times, I drag out a memory (or an armful of memories) and focus on them. I then put them back. The room is a large one. I never lock the door.

Diabetes Kills.

Type 2 Diabetes (mellitus) was the root of all the problems that terminated an energetic, productive life way too early. It directly caused neuropathy that paralyzed her. It slowly and insidiously caused damage to small blood vessels in her brain that led to strokes and TIAs. These damaged blood vessels in her brain also generated the dementia that was probably the hardest thing for both of us to handle.

Everyone should know that the complications from Type 2 Diabetes can be the following:

- Eye problems, including trouble seeing (especially at night), and light sensitivity. Blindness can occur.
- Feet and skin can develop sores and infections and potentially amputation.
- Diabetes may make it harder to control blood pressure and cholesterol. This can lead to a heart attack, stroke, and other problems. It can become harder for blood to flow to your legs and feet.
- <u>Nerves can get damaged,</u> causing pain, tingling, and a loss of feeling.
- High blood sugar can lead to <u>kidney damage</u>. Your kidneys may not work as well, and they may even stop working.

Funeral home/director.

The handling of the administrative and logistical tasks related to giving your loved one the deserved and proper respect and dignity after death is more numerous than you can imagine. It is imperative that you engage the services of a professional in this regard.

A good funeral director (and we had one) lifts a huge burden from your shoulders. You are then free to focus on the real matter at hand. That real matter is to lead your family (and hers) through a very difficult time. Celia still mattered most. We all gathered in several places over time and grieved in various ways —sometimes in a group and sometimes alone. But we were always able to maintain an even keel because we knew that the details and necessities were being handled effectively and efficiently. There are a myriad of legal and governmental issues that need to be handled, some of them with some short deadlines. This is where the professional funeral staff excels. Death certificates were prepared, social security notifications were made, and obituaries were published. I was surprised to learn that as her surviving spouse, I was entitled to continue receiving a portion of Celia's monthly social security payment until I reached eligibility for my own social security benefits.

Feeding the bureaucracy.
You will need to inform a number of organizations of what has transpired. The funeral director will have handled the legally required notifications to local authorities and major federal entities. In our case, the Social Security Administration, the Veterans

Administration, and the local governmental authorities were advised of Celia's passing.

You will need a number of original copies of the death certificate. It is issued by a governmental body that can vary by location. In Nevada it is issued by the State Registrar of Vital Statistics. In other places it is issued by a municipal court.

Assuming life insurance exists, the insurance company will need an original death certificate be submitted together with a package of financial forms. Many insurance carriers now pay proceeds by establishing an interest-bearing account with checking access.

Celia was a retired federal worker. I informed by phone the Office of Personnel Management (OPM) in Washington, DC, of her passing. They sent a packet of forms to complete and return with another original death certificate. The surprising lesson I learned here was that Celia's retirement pay, health insurance, and a small life insurance policy all accrued to me. I had expected that the health insurance might be something I could continue on a paid basis. I had no idea that I had survivor's rights to a portion of her actual retirement stipend and to a cash payment based on her years of federal service and her salary at the time of her retirement. Sometimes feeding the bureaucracy can feed you back.

Afterword

She has gone to a better place. I am certain that she is glad to be there. I am also glad that her suffering has ended and she is now in a place of rest and peace.

I do now feel some relief from having told this story. I did watch my wife die over a long period. I did everything to support her physical, mental, and emotional health that I could. I did ensure that she received every form of dignity and respect that I could imagine.

I can only hope that this story will be of some help to those of you who read it.

In 1969 Stanley Kubrick released a very popular movie called *2001: A Space Odyssey*. The final scene of that movie was a silent image of a large globe (presumably the earth). Upon closer examination, however, one saw that the earth's landmasses and oceans actually formed an almost subliminal outline of a human fetus. That image became the basis of many differing opinions about its meaning. I always thought that it meant that the only thing that could possibly follow the end of something is a new beginning for something else.

I am now even more convinced that my thoughts in 1969 were spot-on. Celia's life on earth has ended. Mine has not. Scott, Sean, Alexandra, Ellie, and Kayli are alive, healthy, and (most importantly) young. The only thing that could possibly follow the end of Celia's life is a newly restarted life for those of us who remain.

THE MOURNER'S BILL OF RIGHTS

Though you should reach out to others as you do the work of mourning, you should not feel obligated to accept the unhelpful responses you may receive from some people. You are the one who is grieving, and as such, you have certain "rights" no one should try to take away from you.

The following list is intended both to empower you to heal and to decide how others can and cannot help. This is not to discourage you from reaching out to others for help, but rather to assist you in distinguishing useful responses from hurtful ones,

1. You have the right to experience your own unique grief.

No one else will grieve in exactly the same way you do. So, when you turn to others for help, don't allow them to tell what you should or should not be feeling.

2. You have the right to talk about your grief.

Talking about your grief will help you heal. Seek out others who will allow you to talk as much as you want, as often as you want, about your grief. If at times you don't feel like talking, you also have the right to be silent.

3. You have the right to feel a multitude of emotions.

Confusion, disorientation, fear, guilt and relief are just a few of the emotions you might feel as part of your grief journey. Others may try to tell you that feeling angry, for example, is wrong. Don't take these judgmental responses to heart. Instead, find listeners who will accept your feelings without condition.

4. You have the right to be tolerant of your physical and emotional limits.

Your feelings of loss and sadness will probably leave you feeling fatigued.

Respect what your body and mind are telling you. Get daily rest. Eat balanced meals. And don't allow others to push you into doing things you don't feel ready to do.

5. You have the right to experience "grief bursts."

Sometimes, out of nowhere, a powerful surge of grief may overcome you. This can be frightening, but is normal and natural. Find someone who understands and will let you talk it out.

6. You have the right to make use of ritual.

The funeral ritual does more than acknowledge the death of someone loved. It helps provide you with the support of caring people. More importantly, the funeral is a way for you to mourn. If others tell you the funeral or other healing rituals such as these are silly or unnecessary, don't listen.

7. You have the right to embrace your spirituality.

If faith is a part of your life, express it in ways that seem appropriate to you.

Allow yourself to be around people who understand and support your religious beliefs. If you feel angry at God, find someone to talk with who won't be critical of your feelings of hurt and abandonment.

8. You have the right to search for meaning.

You may find yourself asking, "Why did he or she die? Why this way? Why now?" Some of your questions may have answers, but some may not. And watch out for the clichéd responses some people may give you. Comments like, "It was God's will" or "Think of what you have to be thankful for" are not helpful and you do not have to accept them.

9. You have the right to right to treasure your memories.

Memories are one of the best legacies that exist after the death of someone loved. You will always remember. Instead of ignoring your memories, find others with whom you can share them.

10. You have the right to move toward your grief and heal.

Reconciling your grief will not happen quickly. Remember, grief is a process, not an event. Be patient and tolerant with yourself and avoid people who are impatient and intolerant with you. Neither you nor those around you must forget that the death of someone loved changes your life forever.

By Alan D. Wolfelt, PhD

The Center for Loss and Life Transition

3735 Broken Bow Road, Fort Collins, CO 80526

www.centerforloss.com

Arlington National Cemetery Burial Eligibility

As of: June 2011

Eligibility for Interment (Ground Burial)

The persons specified below are eligible for ground burial in Arlington National Cemetery. The last period of active duty of former members of the Armed Forces must have ended honorably. Interment may be casketed or cremated remains.

    a.   Any active duty member of the Armed Forces (except those members serving on active duty for training only).

b. Any veteran who is retired from active military service with the Armed Forces.

c. Any veteran who is retired from the Reserves is eligible upon reaching age 60 and drawing retired pay; and who served a period of active duty (other than for training).

d. Any former member of the Armed Forces separated honorably prior to October 1, 1949 for medical reasons and who was rated at 30% or greater disabled effective on the day of discharge.

e. Any former member of the Armed Forces who has been awarded one of the following decorations:
    1. Medal of Honor
    2. Distinguished Service Cross (Navy Cross or Air Force Cross)
    3. Distinguished Service Medal
    4. Silver Star
    5. Purple Heart

f. The President of the United States or any former President of the United States.

g. Any former member of the Armed Forces who served on active duty (other than for training) and who held any of the following positions:
    1. An elective office of the U.S. Government
    2. Office of the Chief Justice of the United States or of an Associate Justice of the Supreme Court of the United States.

3. An office listed, at the time the person held the position, in 5 USC 5312 or 5313 (Levels I and II of the Executive Schedule).

4. The chief of a mission who was at any time during his/her tenure classified in Class I under the provisions of Section 411, Act of 13 August 1946, 60 Stat. 1002, as amended (22 USC 866) or as listed in State Department memorandum dated March 21, 1988.

h. Any former prisoner of war who, while a prisoner of war, served honorably in the active military, naval, or air service, whose last period of military, naval or air service terminated honorably and who died on or after November 30, 1993.

i. The spouse, widow or widower, minor child, or permanently dependent child, and certain unmarried adult children of any of the above eligible veterans.

j. The widow or widower of:

1. a member of the Armed Forces who was lost or buried at sea or officially determined to be missing in action.

2. a member of the Armed Forces who is interred in a US military cemetery overseas that is maintained by the American Battle Monuments Commission.

     3. a member of the Armed Forces who is interred in Arlington National Cemetery as part of a group burial.

  k. The surviving spouse, minor child, or permanently dependent child of any person already buried in Arlington National Cemetery.

  l. The parents of a minor child, or permanently dependent child whose remains, based on the eligibility of a parent, are already buried in ANC. A spouse divorced from the primary eligible, or widowed and remarried, is not eligible for interment.

  m. Provided certain conditions are met, a former member of the Armed Forces may be buried in the same grave with a close relative who is already buried and is the primary eligible.

Eligibility for Inurnment in the Columbarium

The following persons are eligible for inurnment in the Columbarium. The last period of active duty (other than for training) of former members of the Armed Forces must have ended honorably.

  a. Any member of the Armed Forces who dies on active duty.

  b. Any former member of the Armed Forces who is retired from active duty.

  c. Any former member of the Armed Forces who served on active duty (other than for training).

  d. Any member of a Reserve Component of the Armed Forces who dies while he/she is..

1. On active duty for training or performing full-time service under Title 32, United States Code.
2. Performing authorized travel to or from that duty or service.
3. On authorized inactive duty training including training performed as a member of the Army National Guard or the Air National Guard (23 USC 502).
4. Hospitalized or being treated at the expense of the United States for injury or disease incurred or contracted while he/she is on that duty or service, performing that travel or inactive duty training, or undergoing that hospitalization or treatment at the expense of the United States.

e. Any member of the Reserve Officers' Training Corps of the Army, Navy, or Air Force whose death occurs while he/she is...
1. Attending an authorized training camp.
2. On an authorized practice cruise.
3. Performing authorized travel to or from that camp or cruise.
4. Hospitalized or receiving treatment at the expense of the United States for injury or disease incurred while attending camp or cruise, performing that travel, or receiving that hospitalization

or treatment at the expense of the United States.

f. Any citizen of the United States who, during any war in which the United States has been engaged, served in the Armed Forces of any government allied with the United States during that war; whose last service ended honorably by death or otherwise; and who was a citizen of the United States at the time of entry into that service and at the time of death.

g. Certain commissioned officers of the National Oceanic and Atmospheric Administration (formerly United States Coast and Geodetic Survey).

h. Certain commissioned officers of the US Public Health Service.

i. Spouses and minor and certain adult children of those eligible above.

j. Any person eligible for ground burial.

k. A former member of a group that has been certified as active military service for the purpose of receiving VA benefits under the provisions of Section 401, Public Law 95-202.

Source: http://www.arlingtoncemetery.mil/ funeral_information/

Pallas Athene Insignia & Goddess

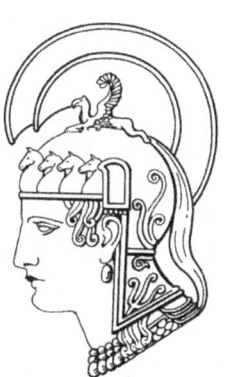

The image above was part of the estate of Brigadier General Elizabeth Hoisington who was the Director of the US Army Women's Army Corps from 1966 to 1971.

Pallas Athene was selected as the insignia of the Women's Army Corps when designers from the Heraldic Section of the Quartermaster General's Office, Headquarters, Department of the Army,

> ... hit upon the idea of a head of Pallas Athene, a Roman and Greek Goddess associated with an impressive variety of womanly virtues...She was the goddess of handicrafts, wise in industries of peace and arts of war, also the goddess of storms and battle, who led through victory to peace and prosperity. Accordingly, the head of Pallas Athene, together with the traditional US, was selected for lapel insignia, cut out for officers and on discs for enlisted women.

Pallas Athene constitutes a strong reference to Mount Olympus and her various Greek and Roman mythological attributes —emphasizing her role as goddess of wisdom, contemplation, handicrafts, the professions, the arts, and war, but most of all her civic duties as guardian of the household.

The name Pallas characterized the goddess as the brandisher of lightning and often her Palladium, or sacred image, holds the brandished lance high in the air. As goddess of storms and thunderbolts, she was called Pallas Athene. Her Latin name, Minerva is connected with the Sanskrit, Greek, and Latin words for mind. (The WAC's affectionately called her "Minnie"). At birth Athene sprang, full grown and dressed in armor, from the forehead of Zeus, King of the Gods, and represented the intellectual aspects of war.

She was the Goddess who caused people to awake and therefore, the Goddess of Wisdom. As Goddess of Wisdom she pleaded for justice tempered with reason and mercy. She was also patroness of arts and crafts being particularly skilled in spinning and weaving.

- Eldora Engebretson, Women's Army Corps Veterans' Association
- PO Box 5577, Ft. McClellan 36205-5577
- www.armywomen.org

History of the Women's Army Corps

The Beginning

The Honorable Edith Nourse Rogers, Congresswoman from Massachusetts, introduced the first bill to establish a women's auxiliary in May 1941. On 14 May 1942, Congress approved the creation of a Women's Army Auxiliary Corps (WAAC). Two days later, Mrs. Oveta Culp Hobby was appointed the first Director of the WAAC.

Five training centers were opened within a year. The first at Fort Des Moines, Iowa, the second at Daytona Beach, Florida, the third at Fort Oglethorpe,

Georgia, the fourth at Fort Devens, Massachusetts, and the fifth at Camp Ruston, Louisiana. As an auxiliary of the Army, the WAAC had no military status, therefore Mrs. Rogers introduced another bill in 1943 to enlist and appoint women in the Army of the United States. President Franklin D. Roosevelt signed the bill on 1 July 1943 and 90 days later the WAAC was discontinued and in its place was the Women's Army Corps (WAC). Colonel Hobby continued as Director of the WAC.

Overseas in World War II

Six months before women received military status, the first WAAC contingent arrived in Algeria, North Africa. In July 1943, the first WAAC Separate Battalion arrived in England led by Lt. Col. Mary A. Hallaren. Three WAC's joined Vice Admiral Lord Louis Mountbatten's Southeast Asia Command in New Delhi, India, in October 1943. A WAC platoon arrived in Caserta, Italy in November and a month later another arrived in Cairo, Egypt. January 1944 marked the arrival of the first WAC's in the Pacific at New Caledonia. In May a large group arrived in Sydney, Australia.

The End of the War

After Victory in Europe (VE) Day in May 1945 and the surrender of the Japanese in August, the remaining WAC training centers at Fort Oglethorpe and Fort Des Moines closed and no further WAC training was conducted. In February 1946, the War

Department began a program aimed at retaining women still in service and re-enlisting those who had served during World War II. The Chief of Staff General Dwight D. Eisenhower, announced that he would ask Congress to make the Women's Army Corps a part of the Regular Army and the Organized Reserve Corps. By the end of May 1946, WAC strength had dropped from a wartime high of more than 99,000 to about 21,500 and by the end of May 1948, WAC strength totaled approximately 6,500 women on active duty.

Regular Army Status

On 12 June 1948 President Harry S. Truman signed into law the Women's Armed Services Integration Act that permitted women in the Regular Army and the Organized Reserve Corps. A new training Center at Camp Lee, Virginia was opened in July 1948.

The Korean War

With the beginning of the Korean conflict, women were again needed in greater numbers than in peacetime. In August 1950, many WAC Officers and enlisted reservists returned voluntarily on active duty, but when more were needed the Army involuntarily recalled a number of reservists on active duty. New WAC detachments were established in Japan and Okinawa to support the men fighting in Korea. A WAC unit was not sent to Korea, but in 1952, a number of individual women filled administrative positions in Pusan and Seoul.

Establishment of a new WAC Center at Fort McClellan, Alabama

In 1951, Congress appropriated funds to establish a permanent home for the WACs at Fort McClellan, Alabama, and in September 1954 General Matthew B. Ridgeway, Chief of Staff of the Army dedicated the Center. The Center conducted basic training, clerk-typist, stenography, personnel specialist, leadership, and cadre courses for enlisted personnel and basic and advanced courses for officers. The first commander of the WAC Center was Lt. Col. Eleanore C. Sullivan.

Vietnam

The first WAC officer assigned to Vietnam in March 1962 was Major Anne Marie Doering. Two WAC advisors to the Vietnam Women's Army Forces Corps were next to arrive in January 1965 —Lt. Col. Kathleen I. Wilkes and master Sergeant Betty L. Adams. They were replaced annually. A WAC detachment with an average strength of 90 enlisted women was located at HQ, US Army, Vietnam, Long Binh, approximately 20 miles from Saigon. The detachment remained there from January 1967 until October 1972 when all US troops began to withdraw from Vietnam. Many enlisted women and WAC officers also served at General Westmoreland's headquarters in Saigon throughout this same period.

Women Generals

On 8 November 1967 Congress removed promotion restrictions on women officers, making it possible for women to achieve general officer rank. The first WAC officer to be promoted to Brigadier General Elizabeth P. Hoisington on 11 June 1970, the second was Mildred C. Bailey, and the third was Mary E. Clarke. They were the seventh, eighth, and ninth (and last) Directors of the WAC, respectively.

WAC Expansion Begins

A major expansion of the WAC began in 1972 as a means of helping the Army maintain its required strength after elimination of the draft on 30 June 1973. As a result of a strong recruiting campaign and the opening of all Military Occupational Specialties (MOS) to women except those involving combat duties, the strength of the WAC increased from 12,260 in 1972 to 52,900 in 1978.

Innovations in the WAC after 1972

Women entered the Reserve Officer Training Corps (ROTC) beginning in September 1972. By May 1981 approximately 40,000 women were enrolled in college and university ROTC programs. On 1 July 1974 all WAC officers were permanently detailed to other branches of the Army (except the combat arms) and the WAC officers' career branch was reduced to zero. Defensive weapons training for enlisted women, warrant officers and women officers became a mandatory course in July 1975. The policy also applied to women in the Reserve and National Guard. In the fall of 1977, women began taking the same basic training course as enlisted men and a year later they began training together in the same units. After four-year trial period, joint training was discontinued in August 1982. The first women cadets entered the United States Military Academy at West Point in July 1976 and women have graduated with every class since June 1980. To fully utilize barracks space worldwide, separate WAC units were phased out in 1973 and 1974. Enlisted women continued to be housed separately to insure privacy in sleeping and bath facilities, but they are jointly administered by a commander and cadre group. The WAC Center and School closed in December 1976. A home for the Women's Army Corps Museum was constructed at Fort McClellan, Alabama in 1977 with funds donated by WAC personnel and their friends. With the closing of Ft McClellan, a new museum will be built at Ft. Lee, Virginia.

Discontinuance of the Women's Army Corps
As a means of assimilating women more closely into the structure of the Army and to eliminate any feeling of separateness from it, the office of the Director, WAC was discontinued on 26 April 1978. The Women's Army Corps as a separate corps of the Army was disestablished on 29 October 1978 by an Act of Congress.

> – Eldora Engebretson, Women's Army Corps Veterans' Association
> PO Box 5577, Ft. McClellan 36205-5577
> www.armywomen.org

Some Useful Online Resources

American Association of Retired Persons
www.aarp.org

Alzheimer's Association
www.alz.org

American Legion
www.legion.org

Arlington National Cemetery
www.arlingtoncemetery.mil/funeral_information

The US Army Women's Army Corps Association
www.armywomen.org

The Home Nursing and Home Care Foundation
www.caregiving.org

The Diabetes Foundation
www.diabetes.org

Helpguide
www.helpguide.org

The Hospice Foundation
www.hospicefoundation.org

The National Association of Insurance and Financial Advisors
www.naifa.org

The Neuropathy Foundation
www.neuropathy.org

The National Funeral Directors Association
www.nfda.org

The National Medical Library at the National Institutes of Health
www.nlm.nih.gov/medlineplus/ (dementia or stroke or neuropathy)

The Office of Personnel Management
www.opm.gov

The National Stroke Association
www.stroke.org

The US Veterans Administration
www.va.gov

Wikipedia, The Free Encyclopedia
En.wikipedia.org

Acknowledgments

Alan D. Wolfelt, PhD, and the Center for Loss and Life Transition for "The Mourner's Bill of Rights"

The US Army for the
"Arlington National Cemetery Burial Eligibility Criteria"

Eldora Engebretson, Women's Army Corps Veterans' Association for
"Pallas Athene Insignia & Goddess" and "History of the Women's Army Corps"

References

N. Lewis and M. Reinhold, eds. "*Roman Civilization*", 3rd Ed, Columbia, 1990

Edward Cheung, "Baby Boomers, Generation X and Social Cycles: North American Long-waves". Long Wave Press, 2007.

Joan Didion, "The Year of Magical Thinking", Vintage Books/Random House, 2006

Reinhold Niebuhr for "The Serenity Prayer"

Abraham Maslow, *A Theory of Human Motivation, Psychological Review*, 1943,

I.A. Richards, The Meaning of Meaning: A Study of the Influence of Language upon Thought and of the Science of Symbolism. Co-authored with C. K. Ogden. London and New York, 1923.